green mama-to-be

green mama-to-be

Creating a Happy, Healthy, and Toxin-Free Pregnancy

Manda Aufochs Gillespie

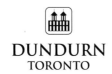

DUNDURN
TORONTO

Printer: Friesens

Front cover images: Vanessa Filley (top left, bottom left, bottom right); Roxanne Engstrom (top right); istock.com/RuslanDashinsky (centre)

Back cover images: Vanessa Filley

Library and Archives Canada Cataloguing in Publication

Aufochs Gillespie, Manda, author
Green mama-to-be : creating a happy, healthy, and
toxin-free pregnancy / Manda Aufochs Gillespie.

Includes bibliographical references and index.
Issued in print and electronic formats.
ISBN 978-1-4597-3628-3 (softcover).--ISBN 978-1-4597-3629-0
(PDF).--ISBN 978-1-4597-3630-6 (EPUB)

1. Pregnant women--Health and hygiene. 2. Pregnancy--
Environmental aspects. 3. Infants--Care--Environmental
aspects. I. Title.

RG525.A94 2017   618.2   C2017-903410-3
                                       C2017-903411-1

    1   2   3   4   5   21   20   19   18   17

  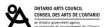

We acknowledge the support of the **Canada Council for the Arts**, which last year invested $153 million to bring the arts to Canadians throughout the country, and the **Ontario Arts Council** for our publishing program. We also acknowledge the financial support of the **Government of Ontario**, through the **Ontario Book Publishing Tax Credit** and the **Ontario Media Development Corporation**, and the **Government of Canada**.

Nous remercions le **Conseil des arts du Canada** de son soutien. L'an dernier, le Conseil a investi 153 millions de dollars pour mettre de l'art dans la vie des Canadiennes et des Canadiens de tout le pays.

Care has been taken to trace the ownership of copyright material used in this book. The author and the publisher welcome any information enabling them to rectify any references or credits in subsequent editions.
— *J. Kirk Howard, President*

The publisher is not responsible for websites or their content unless they are owned by the publisher.

Printed and bound in Canada.

VISIT US AT

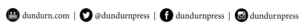

dundurn.com | @dundurnpress | dundurnpress | dundurnpress

Dundurn
3 Church Street, Suite 500
Toronto, Ontario, Canada
M5E 1M2

This book is dedicated to our grandchildren
and all of the future generations. May we pass on to
you a green planet and the most healthy, happy,
and free parts of ourselves.

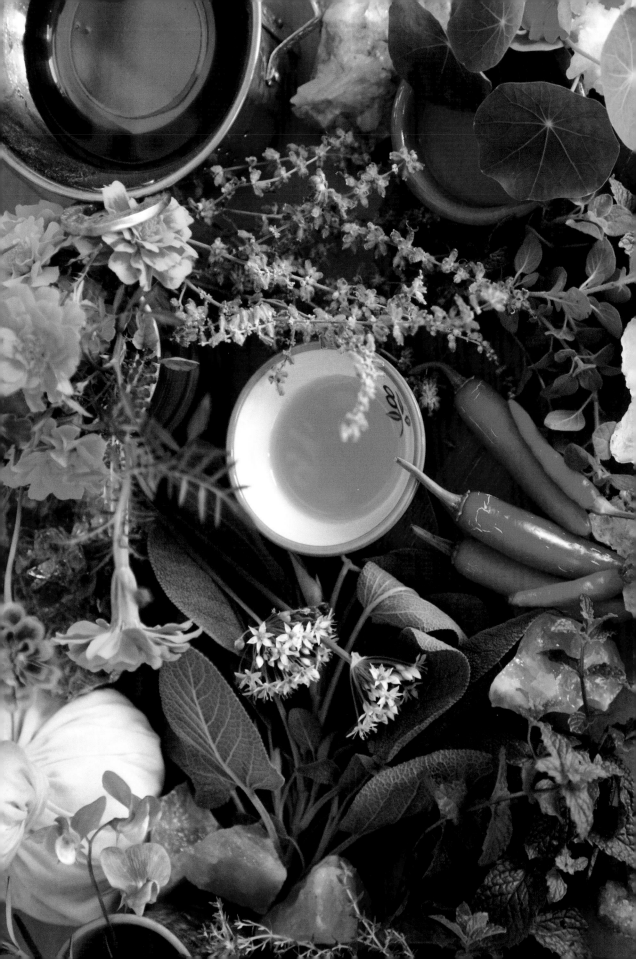

Contents

Introduction

• •

A good farmer farms soil. The plant grows itself.

This saying sums up my experience of parenting. At our best, parents are just good farmers, preparing that soil of family, rhythm, meals, and home from which our children are nourished and fed. This is never more obvious than when the child is still in the womb: where the entire environment of this new life exists within our bodies. Yet pregnancy is just a preparation for the same truths that we will encounter again and again in child-rearing.

When you choose to be a green parent, you are committing to be that farmer, growing the seeds of beloved new beings by lovingly tending to the soil. You try your best, looking to help from the research, traditional wisdom, and other farmers, but you also come to understand that there is a lot of faith involved, since much of parenting, like farming, is out of your hands.

I must admit, I have forgotten many of the details of my pregnancies. At the time, I thought I never would; but, actually, I'm not all that surprised. Pregnancy was not what I expected. I'd read books and articles and researched many topics, so it wasn't *not* what I expected either; it's just that I truly didn't believe any of it would happen to me — especially the less pleasant stuff.

I've met a lot of parents-to-be over the years through my writing, teaching, and consulting as The Green Mama, and I've come to think that this attitude is ubiquitous — this overwhelming, almost delusional optimism. Having a baby is hope made manifest. The shadow side of hope, however, is a sort of "but that won't be me" attitude that can apply to almost everything, even as it's actually happening to you. For me, this included *I won't be … nauseated, exhausted, incapable of getting out of bed, dry-heaving at the smell of the kitchen, vomiting at the thought of food....* I even thought I wouldn't find birth all that painful or the postpartum period depressing. *Not me.* I'd also told myself I wouldn't gain more than a pound a week. But when my day-by-day pregnancy guide said, "You may

The Crib Sheet

Confused by an acronym in the book? Here they are spelled out.

AAP American Academy of Pediatrics

ADHD attention deficit/hyperactivity disorder

AMA American Medical Association

BPA bisphenol-A and **BPS**: bisphenol-S (both are plasticizers)

CDC United States Centers for Disease Control and Prevention

CFL compact fluorescent light bulb

CMA Canadian Medical Association

CPS Canadian Paediatric Society

C-section Caesarean section

DDT dichlorodiphenyltrichloroethane (a pesticide: DDE and DDD are similar)

DHA and EPA docosahexaenoic acid and eicosapentaenoic acid, found in omega-3 fatty acids

DOHaD Developmental Origins of Health and Disease

DIY do-it-yourself

EMF electromagnetic field

EPA United States Environmental Protection Agency

EU European Union

FDA United States Food and Drug Administration

GBS Group B strep

IARC International Agency for Research on Cancer

IVF in vitro fertilization

Hotlist Cosmetic Ingredient Hotlist; Canadian legislation

LED light-emitting diode (type of energy-efficient light bulb)

PBDE polybrominated diphenyl ether, a brominated flame-retardant

PCB polychlorinated biphenyl, industrial toxin

PERC	perchlorate, industrial toxin
POP	persistent organic pollutant
PPB	parts per billion
PPD	postpartum depression
PPD	1,4-paraphenylenediamine and **PTD** 1,4-toluenediamine (similar chemicals in some hair dye)
PFC	perflourinated compounds, include **PFOA** and **PFOS** toxins used in stain-, water-, and oil-resistant materials
PVC	polyvinyl chloride (vinyl)
SIDS	sudden infant death syndrome
SSRI	selective serotonin reuptake inhibitors
TCM	Traditional Chinese Medicine
TRIS	(2-chloroethyl) phosphate, also known as **TCEP** or **TDCP** (toxic flame-retardants)
VOC	volatile organic compound
WHO	World Health Organization

have gained up to five pounds at this point in your pregnancy," I found I was adding a one in front of the five. I just assumed it was a typo. (It wasn't.) *I will never weigh more than 150 pounds*, I'd thought. Well, I did.

Some authors claimed that near the end of pregnancy all those hormones could even get me feeling sexy. They, however, failed to mention how incredibly difficult sex is when your belly forms an awkward (and clearly too late) chastity belt between you and your partner. The authors recommended trying different positions, but the books didn't illustrate these positions that the authors wanted me to try. (I had figured this was because they were prudes, but then I realized it was because the images would be depressing. Just looking at them would tire a pregnant woman out. Or, just as bad, they would tire her partner out!)

I also read that that during pregnancy I might become more emotional. Well, the books didn't mention that I might find myself calmer and more collected than ever, floating along in relative pregnant bliss, only to turn into a sobbing, hysterical wreck just weeks before the baby was born. Or, if they did mention it, they gave totally inadequate explanations like, "This might be caused by the stresses of becoming a parent and preparing for a new family member …," not

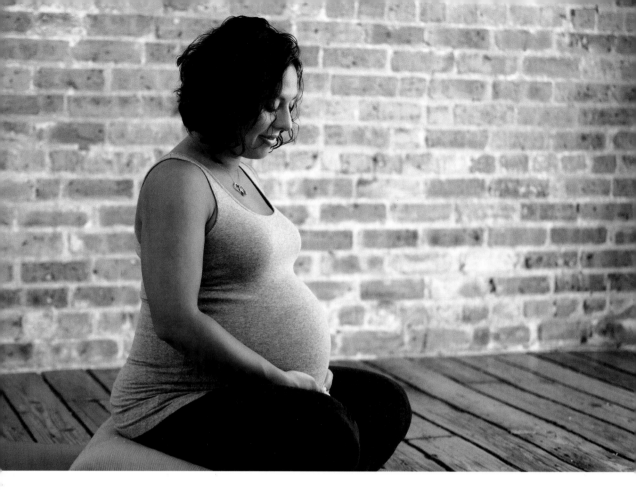

that a two-hour hysterical crying fit might be brought on because my husband came home a half hour late from work or because the sewing machine started sewing backward and refused to go forward (which, of course, would become absolutely, inextricably linked with all my failures as a mother-to-be). They rarely mentioned that there was anything that could be done about it.

I also read that, in preparation for childbirth, my body, which had already nearly doubled its blood volume, would produce more blood, and that it was possible I would experience spontaneous nose bleeds. Okay, fair enough. But, as I found out, when a person gets hysterical over, say, the aforementioned episode in which their husband comes home late (did I mention it was my birthday?), it is possible that they will soak their bed in blood, creating a scene that looks like a reenactment of *The Texas Chainsaw Massacre*.

The bottom line is, there is no book that can completely prepare you for what is to come, and even if it could, you wouldn't believe it.

I've heard childbirth referred to as an experience in which a woman is birthing two new human beings: a baby (or babies) and a mother. This idea is supported by recent discoveries in the field of neuroscience that show that first-time mothers actually grow radically different brains during pregnancy and while caring for their infants. The very biology of parenthood is miraculous, a time when the body grows its only temporary organ (the placenta) and turns the body's stores and consumed food and water into a new being: brain, heart, spine, and tiny feet. I'll never look at dinner the same again.

And when the baby starts to move inside you, the magic and mystery become a conversation. At first it is a conversation spoken in whispers, a language of secrets, dreams, hopes, and expectations. Later, it is a louder conversation in which the demands start emerging: *Feed me! Swim! Rest!* (and, in return, *Get that hand off my bladder please!*) I especially remember that conversation during birth when I suddenly became aware that it wasn't just me labouring to free myself of a baby, but a child labouring to free herself from my ever-tightening womb.

My greatest wish for all new parents is that the act of parenting

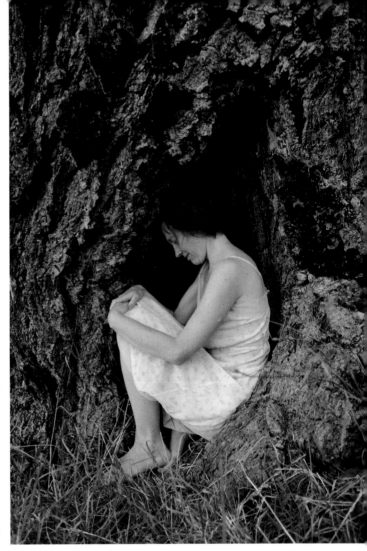

will do that, as well, for you: make you free. Free to be the hopeful, curious, and engaged citizen that makes the act of becoming a parent so powerful. Free to be the expert on the care of your family that you were always meant to be. Free to farm that soil so well that your child, too, will grow up happy, healthy, and free.

How to Make the Most Use of This Book

Read this book however you want — straight through, in sections, or skipping around. You might want to start with the **action steps** that range from the big and bold (♥♥♥) to the easier and more affordable (♥) and the **handbooks** with recipes, tips, and exercises that follow chapters two through seven. You might then take a look at the **inspirational stories** and other **sidebars** and then read the **research** after you have tried out a new action or two. If you like research like I do, you will want to check out the sources and science at the end of the book. If you are low-income or just temporarily broke, don't miss the "**when money matters more**" sidebars.

Today's research adds important details on what is needed to have a healthy, happy, and toxin-free pregnancy in today's world, but the basics are relatively simple and time-tested. Here they are at a glance:

1. Your body and your womb aren't just a blank slate: we will influence our children and our grandchildren by our (hopefully healthy) actions. Our amazing brains will help make our work easier. **Chapter One: Greening the Womb**

2. Our diets are perhaps the biggest source of positive change in shaping our future child's health. **Chapter Two: Greening Your Pregnancy Diet**

3. There are numerous toxins in today's world that we know can have an impact on the health of our developing babies, and there are numerous ways to protect ourselves and our future children *and grandchildren*. **Chapter Three: Greening the Growing Fetus**

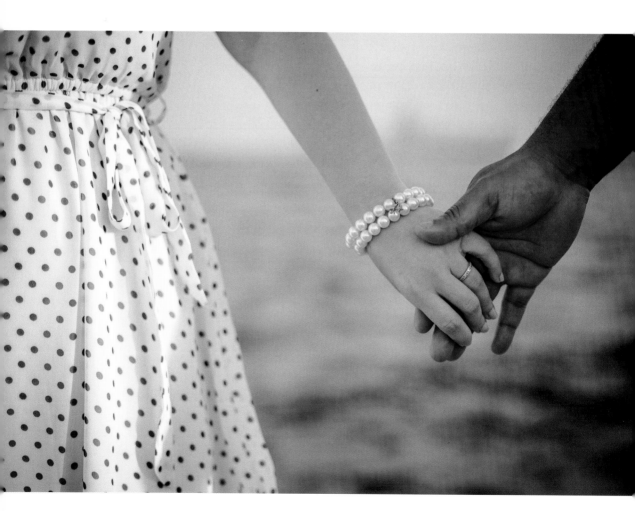

4. Indoor air can be one of our biggest sources of pollution. Luckily it's one of the easiest to clean up. **Chapter Four: Greening Your Home**

5. What goes on the body is as important as what goes in the body. **Chapter Five: Greening Your Beauty Care**

6. Birth and the hour after matter in the life of a family. Set the stage for the healthiest birth, breastfeeding relationship, and first moments of life. **Chapter Six: Greening Birth, Breastfeeding, and Beyond**

7. During the first few months postpartum, a baby has more in common with a fetus than a child. The entire family will benefit from a blissful Fourth Trimester. **Chapter Seven: Greening the Fourth Trimester and Preparing for Postpartum Bliss**

8. How does what you've learned about creating a healthier pregnancy help you make the best choices for your future fertility? The research suggests that diet, toxins, and stress can make a big difference. **Chapter Eight: Greening for Your Future Fertility**

9. If you just want the condensed "cramming for the test" version, skip to the **Conclusion** and the **Green Mama-to-Be*ware*** appendix at the end of the book. While you are there, don't miss recommendations for **Further Reading** and the **Sources**.

This childbearing year is a seed — a tiny blueprint — of what is to come. There are simply endless amounts of research and wisdom that could be shared, but there are also walks in the park, cooking, dreaming, and last dates (without needing a babysitter) to be had, so rather than me writing on and on and you reading on and on, I invite you to bring your specific questions not covered in this book or in *Green Mama: Giving Your Child a Healthy Start and a Greener Future* to me in person or online at www.thegreenmama.com. I look forward to seeing you there.

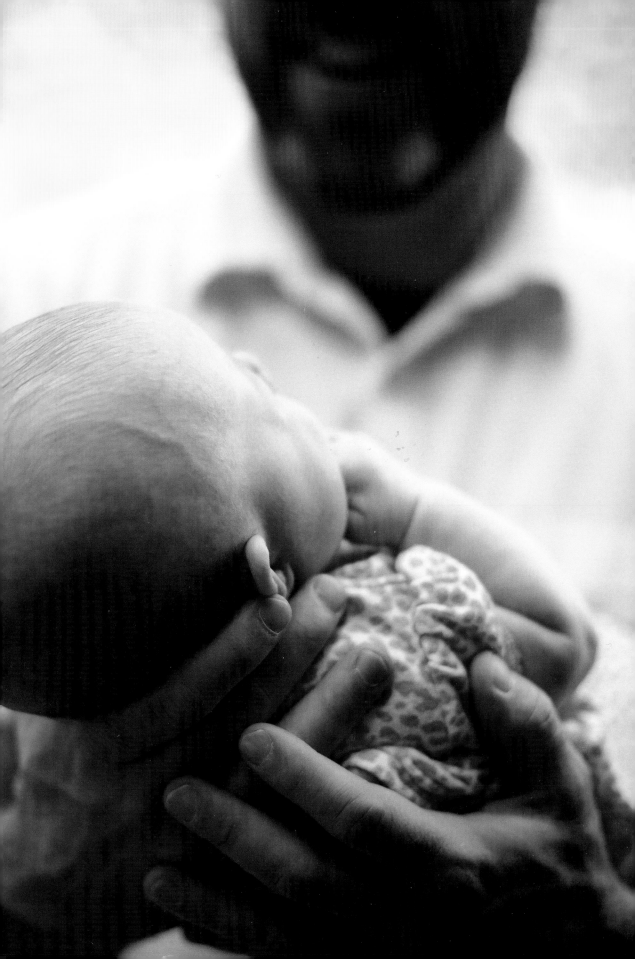

chapter one

Greening the Womb

• •

If you are pregnant right now, you might be surprised to know that you are pregnant not just with your future child, but also with your future grandchildren. Many women know that they are born with all of their eggs, but few realize what this means. Even fewer men realize that their future children are also affected by what happened while they were in their mothers' wombs, and even by their fathers' actions long before conception. In other words, fertility and pregnancy are about the long game: about creating positive change in future generations beyond just your children or even your children's children.

In Traditional Chinese Medicine (TCM), the doctors speak of "heaven" as the moment that conception occurs, and the Pre-heaven Essence is the recognition that the mother and father influence the essence of the child. This Pre-heaven Essence is thought to determine the basic constitution, strength, and vitality of the child, and it is fixed in quantity and determined at birth. It is conserved through life by seeking balance. While that might sound a little woo-woo for some, today's research says something similar in terms of toxins, bacteria, and nutrients: that our children inherit more than just our — and by this I mean both the mother's and father's — genetics, but also some legacy from our lifetime of "environmental" exposures, which includes nutrition, bacteria, toxins, and even stress. To some extent, our children are inheriting these exposures from their grandparents and great-grandparents as well. The exciting thing is that we are able to influence these inheritances; they aren't only predetermined by genetics. Indeed, we are able to have an impact on the future development of our children's genetics during pregnancy even if the children are not genetically our own.

Perhaps the importance of this time leading up to parenthood is why we are also biologically designed to get additional help in the form of hormones and brain changes that make both mothers and fathers better at their new tasks. I loved researching this book because there is simply more research now than there has ever been to explain why your pregnancy is as exciting, emotional, and sometimes as hard as it is: it's truly a time that is as influential as it feels.

The Research

Many women don't realize that they are born with their lifetime supply of eggs. Indeed, a woman reaches her peak number of eggs when she is a fetus between 16 and 22 weeks old. At that time the female ovary contains roughly 6 million immature egg cells (oocytes). By puberty that number is between 100,000 and 400,000, and at menopause only about a thousand remain. With each menstrual cycle, hundreds of oocytes are lost, and one of them matures into an egg, which finds its way into the fallopian tube and starts ovulation. That egg that is eventually formed actually started "waking up" three to four months before ovulation — receiving additional blood flow, nutrition, and oxygen. All in all, the egg is one of the longest-lived cells in the body.

Similarly, even though men produce around 1,500 sperm per second — whether they use them or not — there is a theory that they may be born with a set number of undeveloped seed sperm cells, which mature into active sperm at puberty. Whether this is true or not, a man's supply of sperm is continually replenished throughout adulthood based on the original immature sperm. Spermatogenesis is the process of sperm going from undifferentiated cells in the gonads to mature sperm containing half of the unique genetic information that forms a baby. Spermatogenesis is extremely sensitive to environmental factors such as alcohol intake, tight underwear, and exposure to toxins, heat, and perhaps even electromagnetic fields. Because it takes approximately 70 days and multiple genetic splits for a sperm to mature, there are plenty of opportunities for genetic mutation. Those genes include the chromosome that determines whether the child will be XX (a girl) or XY (a boy).

Most people are aware of the basics of the nature-versus-nurture question: *How much of our children and ourselves is determined by genetics and how much by environment?* For many years most of us — including scientists — thought that the genetics and the environment were in two separate categories: both important, but very different.

Now enter the world of epigenetics, the study of environmental factors that turn genes "on" or "off," determining whether and how genes are expressed. Because epigenetic changes don't affect a person's fundamental DNA, they can be, to some extent, altered by our choices.

For example, one of my friends carried a child using a donated embryo. She found a great deal of comfort in her doctor's advice that she would influence the

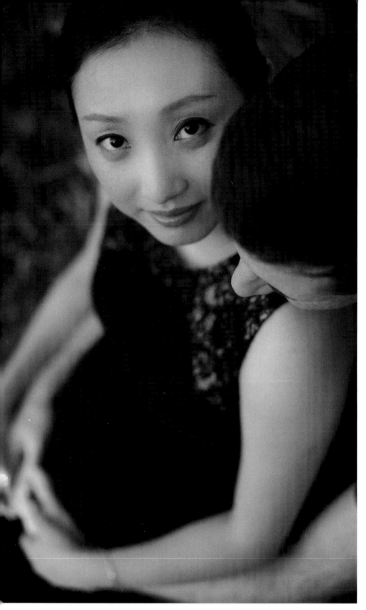

way some of her son's genes would be expressed through her diet, stress levels, environmental exposures, and her own epigenetics. Research into epigenetics confirms that the influence of the womb can begin as early as conception and that what happens in the womb can alter the expression of the growing child's genetics.

Epigenetics Goes Beyond What Happens in the Womb

It doesn't stop, or *start*, there. The changes in those genes can be passed on through the generations. The Överkalix study looked at an isolated community in Sweden from 1890 to 1995. The researchers found that poor food supply could have an effect on mortality, obesity, and diabetes in grandchildren. Most notably, however, it showed that some risks were passed down along sex lines; for instance, if a father started smoking early, it increased the chances of obesity in his sons but not his daughters. Similarly, a grandfather's food availability during the "slow growth period" of eight to twelve years was associated with negative effects in the grandsons but not the granddaughters. A more recent Australian study similarly showed that the sons, but not daughters, of obese fathers were at greater risk of developing obesity, metabolic disorders, and diabetes, even when those children ate the same foods as males whose fathers weren't obese.

In addition, a father's exposure to toxins, such as cigarettes and alcohol, prior to insemination is associated with physical and behavioural changes in the resulting child. Alcoholic fathers are more likely to have children with hyperactivity and reduced cognitive effects. Certain endocrine disruptors can also have effects down the line. The fungicide Vinclozolin — used on the oilseed rape and other fruits and

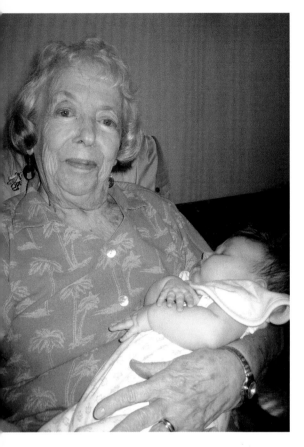

vegetables and considered "not acutely toxic" — has been shown to cause problems in offspring if the father is exposed during critical periods of his own development. In rat studies of this fungicide, males exposed late in their fetal development have sons with an increased risk of tumours, kidney disease, immune system abnormalities, and infertility for at least four subsequent generations through the male line.

Epigenetics and Diet: What Generation of Pottenger's Cats Are You?

I like the story of Dr. Francis Pottenger and his cats as an example of epigenetics: specifically how diet can change the expression of genes. Pottenger studied the health of more than 900 cats over four generations based on diet. He fed one group cooked meat and pasteurized dairy, typical of dried cat food. He fed the other group a healthy diet closer to what they might find in nature, including organ meats and raw meat and milk. Then he examined the health, weight, calcium and phosphorus levels, skeletal structures, and dispositions of the cats over ten years. Within three months the first group started experiencing dental degeneration. Things got worse from there: miscarriages, higher infant and maternal mortality, a dramatic increase in skin diseases and allergies, bone deterioration, hypothyroidism, and personality changes. This group died out completely by the fourth generation. Meanwhile, the second group, which ate the raw diet, thrived generation after generation. Pottenger then tried to restore cats of the first group back to optimal health. He could not do this with third-generation cats because they died before they could reproduce. But, starting with cats from the second generation, he could restore the health of the first group by feeding them the diet of raw milk and meat. Pottenger's observations were an early experiment in epigenetics: each new generation was not a clean slate, but seemed to inherit the physical degeneration caused by the nutritionally inadequate diets of the generations that came before them.

While epigenetics brings light to possible problems, it also gives us hope. Which generation of Pottenger's cats are you? Almost certainly we aren't the lucky recipients of four generations of great, wholesome eating. I grew up poor and spent my early childhood eating processed food from a box supplied by the government. My mother faired a bit better because she grew up in a middle-class family at a time when there were far fewer contaminants in the air, water, and food. My grandmother had what came close to an optimal diet, as her family raised most of what they ate and had ready access to fresh eggs and real milk. They also ate very little that was processed. So it seems I am a revival generation, working toward better health for me and my children and aiming for the optimal health of my children's children.

The Role of Bacteria in Genetics

Epigenetics isn't the only new scientific buzzword that is radically changing the way we think about health and inheritance. Now the talk is about the *microbiome*. This refers to an ecological community of microorganisms that share our body space. To begin to understand the idea of the microbiome, it's essential to understand that human bodies contain trillions of bacteria. We have as many bacteria and other microbes making us up as we have our "own" cells. Not only that, but it would seem that at least some of this bacterial life — such as that lining our gastrointestinal (GI) tracts — have coevolved with us and are unique and essential to our health, especially the functions of our immune system. In other words, to be in a state of complete health, a person will have all the elements of their microbiome living in harmony, and that will include all the human cells as well as bacteria and organisms that might be classified as viruses, parasites, or other as yet unidentified microbes. The microbiome of a healthy human gut will be different from that of a healthy rat gut. In fact, the microbiome of one healthy human's gut might be quite different from that of another healthy human's gut. We have similarly unique microbiomes in our mouths and vaginal tracts and on our skin.

We also know that the gut microbiome has been changing over the generations: namely, becoming less diverse. This is assumed to be a bad thing, much like a lack of diversity in nature, where invasive species can cause serious problems. The likely culprit in this loss of diversity is our modern diet, which is higher in fats and simple carbohydrates and lower in fibre than traditional diets. But the research also brings into question our current practice of using antibacterial products (which are found nearly everywhere, from 90 percent of hand soaps to the lining in our shoes) and our overuse of antibiotics. In short, we must have bacteria and other microbes (and lots of them) for human life to exist, and we need them in good balance in order to be healthy.

A Baby Isn't Born a Blank Slate — Genetically or Bacterially

Until very recently, scientists and doctors believed that the womb was a sterile environment and that a child's first exposure to bacteria occurred as they passed through the birth canal and right after they emerged into the world. In the last

Inspiring Mamas: The Five Levels of Healing

Every day Dr. Katie Dahlgren sees miracles happen. Dr. Dahlgren is a naturopathic physician who specializes in autism, chronic illness, and detoxification. Her practice is largely made up of children who are considered incurable: kids who can't speak or play or make eye contact. Yet many of them get better. "I see kids who are nonverbal at the age of five or six who are able to go on and be integrated back into classrooms…. Our neuroplasticity is way greater than we used to believe."

"People can recover," she says, and it is this knowledge that allows her to balance her work with such sick children while also raising three children of her own. This faith in the ability of humans to recover keeps her hopeful. "The current environment with chemical toxins, heavy metals, and EMF exposure is considerably different than anything else we have faced in human evolution."

All of these man-made chemical exposures are happening as part of a larger ecosystem of microbes. Even as we better understand the important role of bacteria in creating healthy human guts and other organ systems, we still know so little about most microbes. Dahlgren points to viruses as an example of microbes that are always evolving and changing and are poorly understood by the medical establishment. "Our bugs are evolving much faster than our medicine," she says, adding that she sees unprecedented resistance to antibiotics and antifungals. It won't be long before we won't be able to treat many of the treatable diseases of today with our current medicines. The microbes have evolved faster than our ability to treat them. "We need to transition from using pharmaceuticals to finding the right balance of flora," she says. Dr. Dahlgren has found success working with the five levels of healing, a concept developed by her mentor, Dr. Dietrich Klinghardt, MD., Ph.D. The five levels, starting at the lowest level and rising, are the physical body, energetic body, mental body, dream body, and spirit body.

"We aren't just physical beings," she says. If there is a significant trauma in the family, it can affect the epigenetics. An example would be studies that show that people who suffered through famine as children have grandchildren with a higher propensity toward certain diseases. "It isn't enough to just look at toxicity or nutrition. You must look at the entire person as a whole." Work on one level — say, the mental body — can penetrate down to help heal things on the level of the energetic body and the physical body. "You have to look at those lower levels … think of it as the soil of the plant. You can't start pruning the higher levels when the roots are dying." To truly treat people, the practitioner must "address the person in every way they are relating to be a human being."

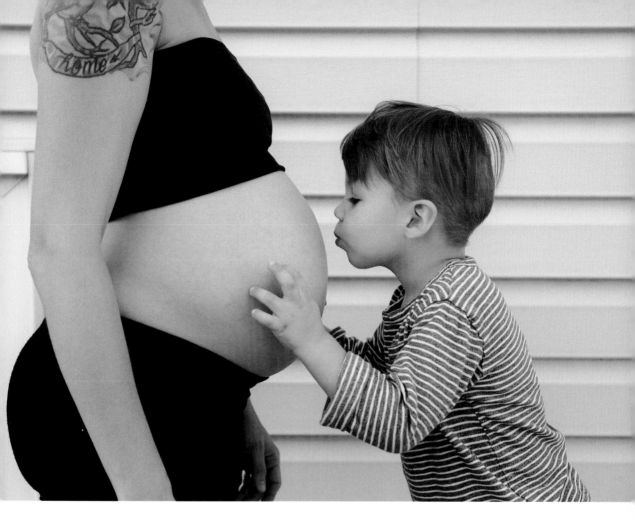

few years, scientists have established that there are bacteria in the amniotic fluid, placenta, meconium (the dark green substance forming the first feces of a new-born infant), and the fetus's intestines, and that the baby's microbiome begins to develop in the womb and is influenced by the mother's health and diet. In particular, there is research to indicate that the developing fetus's microbiome will be affected by his weight at birth as well as by the mother's weight, dental health, and antibiotic use during pregnancy. The baby's microbiome is also dramatically affected by what happens during and immediately after birth — whether it is a vaginal or Caesarean birth, whether there is immediate skin-to-skin contact, and whether the baby is breastfed. These factors are all extremely important in seeding an infant's microbiome.

Aspects of the mother's microbiome can also be passed down to the child and then on to the grandchildren and great-grandchildren through the birth process. In this way, our microbes influence our epigenetics. Although there is still a lot we don't understand about the microbiome and its role over generations, what is clear is that a mother can take steps to ensure the best possible future microbiomes develop in her child, starting before she conceives, during her pregnancy, and throughout her child's life.

Mama (and Papa) Brain: Better Than Ever

The complicated world of the microbiome isn't the only thing we are seeing with new eyes thanks to current scientific research. The amazing world inside our brains is also becoming a bit clearer.

"Pregnancy Brain," "Momnesia," "Mommy-mind": these are all terms that you may understand all too well if you are pregnant while reading this book. That mushy feeling and all the underlying emotions that seem to go along with it during pregnancy are real, and they serve a purpose. Mothers both grow and lose grey matter and their brains get rewired. It's as if the brain is indeed being turned to mush with the help of all those pregnancy and postpartum hormones — oxytocin,

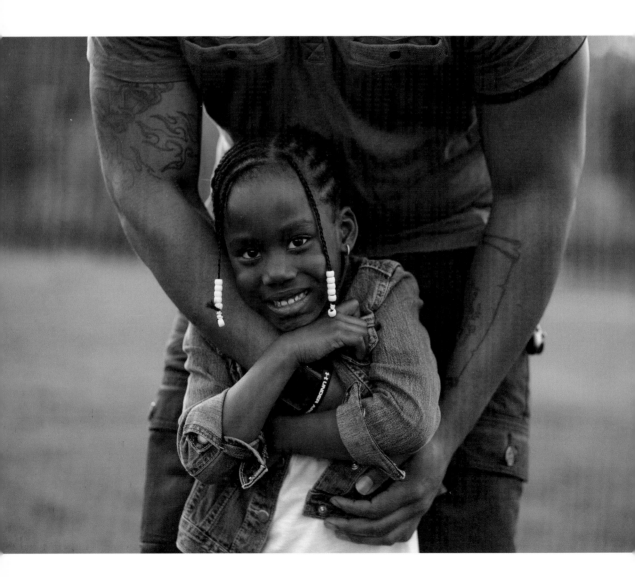

estrogen, prolactin — so that it can be rewired to more effectively perform the work involved in caring for a child. Indeed, many of those so-called pregnancy and postpartum emotions, including love, protectiveness, and even worry, begin in the brain. As with so many aspects of human biology and pregnancy, scientific research into what happens to the brain during pregnancy is revealing massive breakthroughs. Perhaps the science is beginning to catch up to what mothers already know: those brain changes aren't just in our heads.

In December 2016 a new study came out, and the headlines all blared some version of "Pregnancy Shrinks Brains." I found this particularly interesting because a few years earlier the result of another study had prompted headlines that screamed "Pregnant Moms Grow New Brain."

What gives? I wondered.

Both studies showed that first-time mothers consistently demonstrated a notable difference in grey matter volume in parts of their brains. The older study — which showed an increase in grey matter to be associated with the better-adjusted new mother — was complemented by the new study — which showed a positive correlation with a decrease in grey matter — by demonstrating the increases and decreases were in different parts of the brain. The better-adjusted new mothers had increases in parts of the brain that included the prefrontal cortex, amygdala, and the hypothalamus, which is associated with emotional regulation, survival instincts, and hormone production. If these latter areas shrank instead of grew, the result was mothers with more stress, anxiety, and poorer experiences of mothering.

The new study showed that mothers with the best attachments had a decrease in medial frontal and posterior cortex lines that are involved in social cognition, which is how we process, store, and apply information about other people and social situations. The researchers surmised that this period is one of great synaptic pruning, similar to what happens in a young child and again in adolescents, where underused neurological pathways — synapses — are eliminated to make way for new neural networks. The researchers found no corresponding changes in memory or other cognitive functions.

Of particular interest to many researchers was what happens in the amygdala, the part that the old study said ought to grow and that helps process memory and governs emotional reactions such as aggression, anxiety, and fear. In most mothers' brains, this area continues to grow in the weeks and months after giving birth and is full of receptors for that cocktail of hormones that help feed the love, attachment, and care between mother and baby. It's the part of the brain that lights up when the mother stares at her baby or elicits one of those early smiles. If that part of the brain is damaged or not growing normally, the results in the mother are noticeable and can be linked to higher levels of depression and greater anxiety. In the child it may shape whether she can distinguish between her mother and anybody else.

This part of the brain is also particularly sensitive to oxytocin, aka the love hormone, responsible for maternal-infant bonding. Oxytocin dramatically increases in pregnancy and the postpartum period. It also increases with breastfeeding. The more the mother is involved with her child, the greater the increase in oxytocin levels.

Once a Mother, Always a Mother

It is hard to describe how much easier I found adjusting to life after my second child. It felt intuitive, like I had already done most of the work of becoming a mother after having my first. Having the second felt a bit like getting a master's degree: I had already figured out how to be a good student; what was a few more years? Why not spend those years simply worrying less and having more fun, I figured. The brain research backs this up, as the changes in a mother's brain are most dramatic with her first child. Indeed, it isn't clear that the changes ever fully convert. Some researchers explain that it is as if all women have the blueprint inside their brains for motherhood.

Papa Brain Is Also Real and Forever

It's not all about the mothers, however. While the newest study on grey matter was quick to point out that fathers don't grow new brains, other research shows that dads have the capacity for significant brain changes to support parenting. For men, these brain changes don't seem to be driven by oxytocin, but are directly tied to care-giving. The more involved the father, the more he is supported by a feedback loop that helps wire his brain for that involvement.

Interestingly, it's also been found that the "male" hormone testosterone decreases after a man becomes a father, and the more involved he is in childcare, the lower his testosterone drops. This is irrespective of how high his testosterone was before becoming a parent; indeed, men with higher testosterone before parenthood actually seem to have a better chance of becoming fathers. Lower lifetime testosterone may have an impact on men's health, even decreasing the chances of prostate cancer. This, as with much about parenting and the brain, is still being studied, as is whether testosterone levels eventually rebound. This hormonal change, according to some researchers, suggests that men are also preprogrammed to be involved parents.

How to Green the Womb

There is a saying that environmentalists like to quote. It is inspired by the Constitution of the Iroquois Nations: "In every deliberation, we must consider the impact on the seventh generation." Having a child makes the abstract concept of future generations real. Today's science reveals that these ancient traditions are based on our biology: we carry more than just our children in our wombs; we also carry our children's children.

Here are a series of action steps listed from ♥♥♥ (biggest impact, and possibly more work) to ♥ (quick and easy) to help you green your womb for your child and for future generations.

1. ♥♥♥ If you are reading this book before getting pregnant, consider doing a preparatory period (up to a year) to enhance the health of you and your partner. Many fertility researchers suggest that this is even more important for the man. The first step is to ensure you are both digesting well. Then, you might consider undertaking a more intensive cleanse with the help of a nutritionist. And then both of you can begin to eat, drink, and live as if you are already nourishing a new life. Ideally, this nourishing phase would start at least three months before conception. The rest of this book will help!

2. ♥♥ If you have just received this book as a "Congratulations, you're pregnant!" present, that's perfect. Remember, everything you do now will help you, your baby, and your future grandchildren.

3. ♥ It's not just in your head. Brain changes, for mamas and involved partners, are real and specifically designed to help you become the best parent you can be. To help these brain changes, you will learn more about eating for brain health in this book. You will also benefit from the tips on de-stressing, de-cluttering, and simplifying in advance of the baby's arrival.

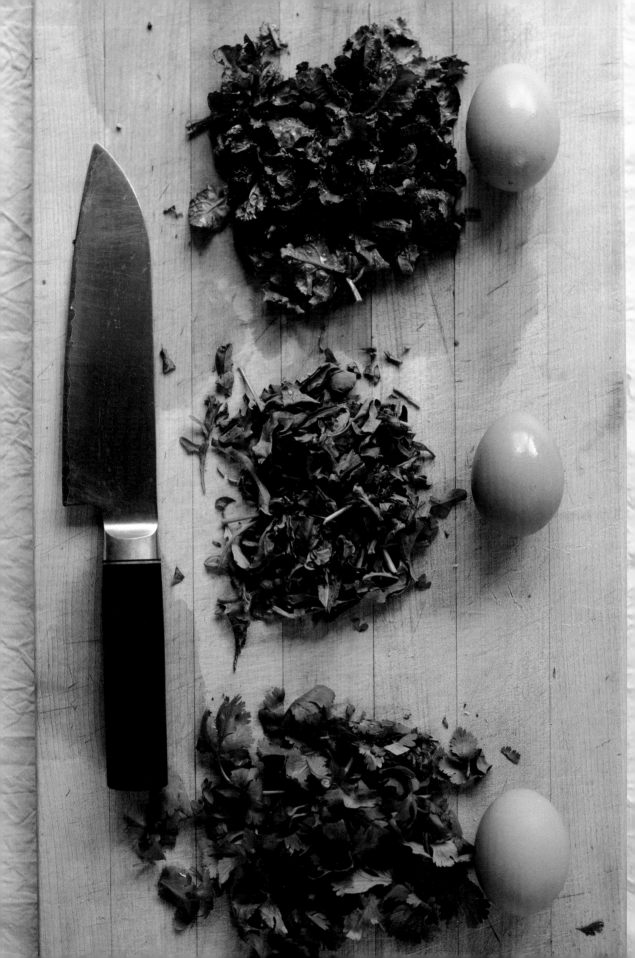

Greening Your Pregnancy Diet

· ·

The body and brain of a child growing in utero are fuelled by nutrients. These nutrients come from the mother's tissues or from her daily intake of food and drink. These nutrients build the baby and provide for the physical changes within the mother's body: growing the placenta and doubling the volume of blood. While this may be completely obvious, it continually amazes me to realize the magnitude of this basic biology. Not only are you what you eat; your baby is too. In addition, evolution put your baby first in line at the buffet. That means the baby will get what he needs from the nutrients you consume and even draw on your reserve stores of protein, healthy fats, calcium, and other nutrients. Thus, a mother can suffer from health problems related to lack of nutrients, even if the child does not. Nutritional deficits can plague women for a lifetime after having their babies and can become a problem in future pregnancies, especially if a woman's nutritional stores are increasingly depleted. The nutrients that a woman consumes to help grow a baby and maintain her own optimal nutrition should be abundant, of high quality, and easily absorbed. These nutrients, after all, make up the blood, tissue, bones, brain, and other organs of our bodies and that of the baby-to-be.

Not all food is created equal, and not all of our bodies are equally able to make use of the nutrients we consume. Refined and fried foods, processed sugars, and food additives don't just fail to nourish; they can actually rob a body of precious nutrients. Similarly, foods that contain pesticides, synthetic hormones, or other environmental toxins can interfere with the body's ability to absorb and use the nutrients in the food itself. And if a woman isn't digesting well, then she won't be able to make full use of the nutrients she does eat.

So how do we grow healthy babies while maintaining a mother's health and restoring it after the birth? It's not as hard as it may seem.

What We Wish Our Grandmothers Had Told Us About Eating for Two

When my grandmother was having her children, the medical establishment encouraged women not to gain too much weight during pregnancy. Doctors would even prescribe diet pills to help expectant mothers stay slim. The general attitude was that the traditions of the past had gotten it wrong and that eating for two was not scientific. American Medical Association (AMA) vice-president Dr. William Carrington warned at that time that eating too many calories would not help grow a baby, but would be "stored as fat in odd and embarrassing places about the body of the mother." The medical community continued to warn women throughout most of the twentieth century about the harm of gaining too much weight, usually suggesting no more than 15 to 20 pounds (7 to 9 kilograms) was recommended, and often much less. The general sentiment was that the growing fetus was so small that it did not have a great nutritional need. They were wrong.

Today, many people still assume that overweight women don't need to consume as many nutrients because they have more nutrients stored. In fact, the opposite is often the case, with many overweight women actually having considerable nutritional deficiencies. Obesity is not a state of being over-nourished, but rather a risk factor for nutritional deficiencies, particularly in many of the antioxidants and fat-soluble vitamins. Studies done on donor eggs show that the obesity factor is not so much genetic as epigenetic: these studies found that the birth weight of the baby was not correlated with anything of the donor's, but rather with the weight of the mother who carried the child. Obese mothers are more likely to have underweight and undernourished babies, who are more likely to go on to be overweight themselves. Some scientists speculate that undernourished babies are born "hungry," as if their metabolism thinks it was born into a world of scarcity, and thereby get more efficient at storing fats and hoarding calories.

Thank goodness that many doctors, midwives, and pregnancy books today are far less fixated on total weight gain, and many are actively supportive of good nutrition. Even in the few years between my first and second pregnancies, I noticed a subtle shift in attitudes. I almost never even weighed myself with my second, while with my first I was nervous about the 45 pounds I had gained. I was extremely grateful, however, for every one of those extra pounds by the time I got to six months postpartum. By then, I weighed less than I had before I had gotten pregnant and was working hard to eat enough while I felt my remaining fat supplies literally being sucked out of me. My friend who had her baby at the same time was a little older than me, and she found she didn't lose that final "five pounds" until after she stopped nursing. Then, she lost it with ease, and she regretted the worry she had carried with her for the past two years.

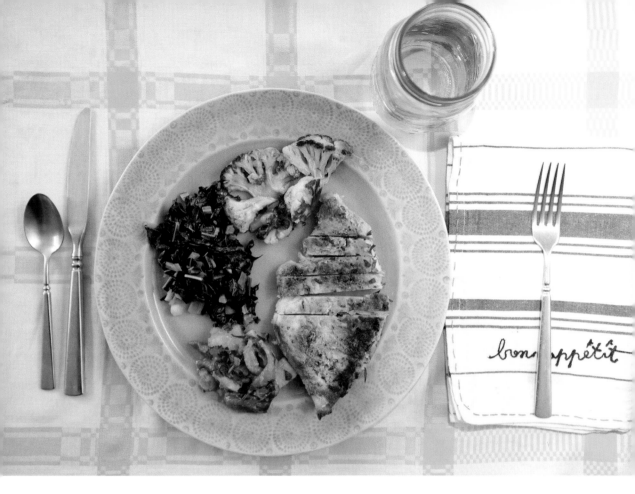

Unfortunately, too many doctors, midwives, and pregnancy books still focus on the total weight gain or the long list of "Don't Eats," rather than on the more significant nutritional needs of nourishing another living being. I've always found the Don't Eat lists to be questionable from both a scientific and an anthropological perspective. How can a good raw cheese and a glass of wine with dinner be such an awful dietary choice for North American women when our French counterparts are told it is fine to have both? Luckily, there is a growing field of science and medicine focused specifically on what composes the best nutrition for health, including for growing a healthy baby.

The Research

There is an entire field of science developing that studies the connection between the nutrition of the baby-to-be in the womb and the connection to chronic disease in adulthood and into future generations. The Developmental Origins of Health and Disease (DOHaD) studies how the months of pregnancy — and the conditions encountered while in the mother's womb — lay the foundation of the immune system and shape the wiring of the baby's brain, the function of the organs, and the child's metabolism. Dr. David Barker initiated this field of science three decades ago with his research linking chronic diseases in adulthood to low birth weights.

Your mother's nutrition during pregnancy (and now yours) is one of the most important indicators of future health. As the organization Better the Future puts it, "Nutrients flow across generations…. This means that a woman's nutrition directly affects not only her own child's health, but her grandchild's health as well."

Despite this rapidly developing field, most doctors today are taught very little about nutrition. Only 27 percent of medical schools in the United States offered the recommended 25 hours of nutritional training, according to a 2010 government report. Fortunately, there is a growing movement of doctors, nutritionists, and other healthcare providers who take an integrative approach to health and nutrition through science, case study, and diet. Known as "functional medicine," this approach focuses on conscientiously supporting the body with the nutrients it needs to keep it in tip-top working condition; in other words, using food as the first line of treatment.

Good Eating Can Be Simple

Margaret Floyd Barry is a functional nutritionist, mother of two, and author of the Eat Naked series of books. Margaret is one of my favourite sources on nutrition because she so thoroughly combines traditional wisdom and current science. She has also learned how to apply this to her own life while running a business and juggling the needs of a preschooler and a nursing child. Her website, www.eatnakednow.com, provides resources for finding a functional nutritionist in your area or working directly with Floyd Barry.

According to her, "the most important thing for pregnancy is that the woman is eating a really nutrient-rich diet the entire time." Eating healthy doesn't have to be hard. In traditional societies, or even 200 years ago, people didn't know any of this stuff. They just ate food.

So if you start to get overwhelmed, or if you're getting conflicting advice, go back to the basics: you are in building mode, and the best building materials for babies haven't changed in the long span in which humans have evolved. Nutrient-dense foods are those that contain good fats and good proteins.

Floyd Barry adds that, before a woman starts worrying about denying herself things in pregnancy, she should focus on adding nutrient-rich foods to her diet and getting her digestive system really working. Getting digestion working well can be as simple as balancing your blood sugar through the slow-carb principles explained below and by adding probiotic-rich and healing foods to your diet.

In Floyd Barry's experience, women who are eating and digesting really well naturally eat enough protein (approximately 113 grams with every meal). But they may have to work harder to get enough good fats, and these are particularly important to a developing baby's nervous system. Fatty proteins are the best; lean proteins — low-fat protein powders, protein bars, and low-fat milk — should be avoided.

Animal fats are a great way to get fat-soluble vitamins, such as vitamin A, that help us make use of the protein we eat. When we eat lean proteins with very little fat and fat-soluble vitamins, our body must use stored fat-soluble vitamins to make proper use of the protein. This can lead to significant deficiencies that can affect sex hormones, vision, and the baby's brain and nervous system. When you eat fat with your protein, it not only provides more nourishment, it also tastes better!

"I don't know a pregnant woman who doesn't crave carbs," says Floyd Barry, "so be smart about it." One way to do this is to front-load every *day* and every *meal* with the most important foods: the good fats, the proteins, and the green, leafy stuff. "If you start with a starch, you will crave starches all day long," she cautions.

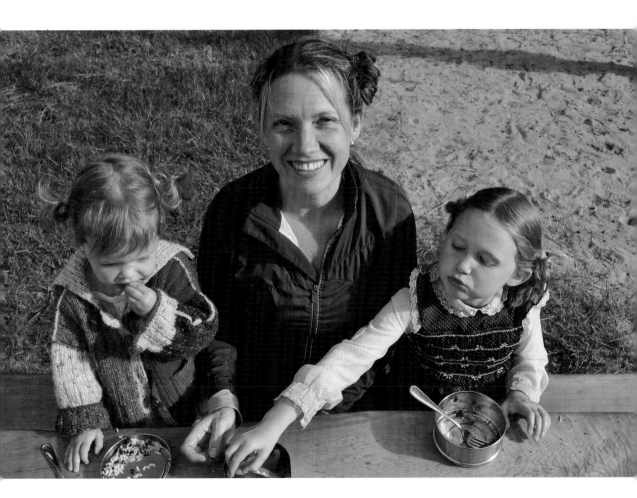

These "slow-carb" principles help mothers-to-be ensure they get the good fats and proteins they need. This includes front-loading the veggies and meats and some legumes and saving small portions of starches — such as a third of a cup of quinoa or half a sweet potato — for the end of the meal. Another trick for pregnancy is to stay in front of the hunger with appropriate fatty-protein snacks such as nuts, cheese, sardines, avocado, bone broth, or nut butter on apple slices (plain fruit as a snack can spike your blood sugar). Check out the **The Green Eating Recipe Handbook**, on pages 64–71, for additional inspiration. Eating foods naturally high in protein and containing good fats, front-loading the good stuff, and enduring snacks follow the same principles will help even out blood sugar levels, improve digestion, and give the baby a steady flow of the nutrients he needs.

Pregnancy is a time to eat nutrient-dense foods; it is not the time to do any sort of cleansing, which includes juice cleanses and strict vegan diets. These kinds of cleanses not only can deny the growing baby important nutrients, but also can cause toxins stored in the mother's body to move through the placenta and into the baby. It's also why Floyd Barry says that "Quality trumps everything else" when eating during pregnancy. You can learn how to source the best-quality animal products, vegetables, fruits, and grains in the **Organic-ize your Diet** section on pages 55–63.

It is also important to properly prepare foods at home: rinsing, soaking, and cooking as needed. No restaurant or manufacturer of packaged food can prepare meals as well and as affordably as you can yourself.

So, what are the most nourishing and healing foods that Floyd Barry recommends you eat during pregnancy? They include organ meats, fish, bone broth, and fermented foods. Foods to further promote good digestion include apple cider vinegar, beet kvass (helps with fat digestion; see the recipe in the Recipe Handbook), and probiotic drinks like kambucha and yogourt shakes, as well as the aforementioned bone broths and fermented foods.

Focus on adding these foods to your diet and using the above strategies to achieve balance before worrying about denying yourself the occasional milkshake or chocolate-dipped pickle surprise.

How Can I Tell If I'm Digesting Properly?

To assess if you're digesting well, just check out your poop! Good digestion results in excrement that has the consistency of soft-serve ice cream and is a nice chocolate brown colour. (Yes, I do recognize that was gross.) There won't be undigested food bits and it won't be super stinky. It does not require any effort or straining, nor does it require a magic elixir such as fibre or a cup of coffee. It will happen at least once a day — best if it is three times a day, shortly after each meal. And it will require only one wipe.

For optimal digestion, your stomach needs to be acidic. *What?!* You may be thinking that an acidic stomach would make issues of heartburn and acid reflux worse. Not so. These are all actually symptoms of hypochlorhydria, meaning the stomach is not acidic enough. For optimal digestion, the stomach needs to have a pH of about 1.5 to 3 (out of a scale of 0 to 14, seven being neutral and everything under being acidic). The blood, on the other hand, is a bit alkaline, at about 7.4. With too little acid in the stomach, food starts to ferment. This creates gas, indigestion, or sometimes stomach acid that will flow back into your food pipe and lead to gastro-esophageal reflux disease (GERD). Proper stomach acid is essential to make proteins and fats available, maintain energy levels, defend against parasites, and protect against food allergies and certain autoimmune diseases. Stress, antacids, vegan diets, poor diets, age, and certain medications can decrease stomach acid. With so many causes, many adults need help to balance their stomach acid levels. Floyd Barry recommends a few things to try at home before seeking out a functional nutritionist for help:

1. Eat slowly and in a relaxed state.
2. Give yourself time to digest after a meal, such as a leisurely 15-minute walk or a quick rest on the couch.
3. Eat your last meal of the day three hours before you go to bed.
4. Drink a glass of warm water with 1 tablespoon of raw apple cider vinegar before meals (or, if you just can't do it, substitute fresh lemon juice).
5. Follow all the slow-carb principles in the previous section, including front-loading the good fats, proteins, and vegetables at every meal.

Digestion versus Metabolism

Metabolism isn't the same as digestion. Digestion is the process of breaking up the food into its nutritive components, and metabolism is the process by which the cells of your body use the energy they got from the digestive process to fuel the cellular work of the body. The length of time your food takes to go from being eaten to being pooped out has little to do with your rate of metabolism.

The foundation of our metabolism begins in the womb. With the cutting of the umbilical cord starts a process that continues until we die. Our metabolism is composed of both **catabolism** — the breakdown of large molecules to create energy — and **anabolism** — using this energy to build up complex molecules needed for developing new tissue and for healing. Enzymes and their helpers make this happen. They support the metabolism but aren't used up in the process.

When we digest, our bodies break down the food into its basic, and smaller, nutritional components: proteins turn into amino acids; carbohydrates and compound sugars are converted into glucose or dextrose to be made into blood; and fats get turned into fatty acids. These amino acids, fatty acids, and sugars are then circulated in the bloodstream until put to use by the cells, where they join with enzymes, vitamins, and minerals to release energy for immediate use, such as building your tissues, or creating the brain of your growing child, or going into storage for future use. At this point, digestion becomes metabolism — the biochemical processing of the nutrients delivered by way of digestion.

The Gut: Your Second Brain

Digestion and the work of the gastrointestinal (or GI) tract is so important that ancient healing traditions such as Ayurveda and TCM both consider the health of the mind to be inextricably linked to the health of the gut. Indeed, we now know there are millions of neurons that connect the brain to our "second brain," aka the enteric nervous system, which controls the GI system and stretches from the esophagus to the anus. This system not only controls digestion, but also can work in conjunction with the brain in your head to influence physical and mental well-being. This connection is at the heart — or stomach — of why we have terms such as "gut-feeling" and why, when we have an awful row with our partner or a bad day at work, we might feel "sick to our stomach" about it. The gut can also help us feel good. The "feel-good" molecule serotonin, produced in the gut, goes into the blood and can help repair cellular damage in the liver and lungs. A 2006 study suggested that stimulation of the vagus nerve, responsible for automatic body functions such as digestion, can be effective for chronic depression. As well, our GI system plays a central role in our immune health: approximately 70 percent of the cells of our immune system reside in the gut.

Digestion starts in the mouth, and that's why chewing slowly and maximizing saliva contact can be so important. After the food leaves the stomach, it then comes to the next biggest player in the digestive system: the small intestine. The major work of digesting starches, proteins, and fats happens here, with chemical support coming from the liver and pancreas. As the starches, proteins, and fats get broken down, the small intestine absorbs the nutrients into the bloodstream through millions of minuscule hair-like villi that line the intestinal wall. Whatever isn't absorbed into the small intestine passes on to the large intestine, aka the colon, where it is further processed and where water gets absorbed. Whatever is left of what started as food and drink is removed from the colon through defecation.

Our Natural Detoxification Process

These days, everybody has heard of detoxification, even though it's not a concept that my grandmother learned much about in her college's home economics program. Though our world has a growing number of toxins to which we are exposed, toxins aren't new. Indeed, detoxification is just our body's way of cleaning up, and that includes natural processes, such as metabolism. Those used up biochemicals don't just hang around indefinitely, but are broken down and disposed of like your recycling or garbage. Thus, our bodies are busy cleaning up after all the usual aspects of living — eating, exercising, having babies, aging. Plus, we've added all sorts of new toxins to the mix, like recurrent stress, medications, environmental factors, and processed foods. Our body's detoxification system can help with modern pollutants to some extent, but not always. Breakdowns occur when the system gets "gummed up," when the input of toxins increases, or during pregnancy and breastfeeding when our babies receive some of what is being detoxified from our bodies.

The liver is the workhorse of detoxification, and there is a great deal of variability between people in how much and how well their livers can handle detoxification. The liver tries to filter out the junk, such as pesticides, medications, used-up hormones, unnecessary by-products of digestion, and indigestible leftovers like some food additives. As well, the liver meets with many toxins that are inhaled (not just from car exhaust and factories, but also from nail polish and cleaners, or even that new pressed-wood bookcase).

Nutrition can help support the health and effectiveness of the liver and the other organs of detoxification, which include the skin (which I've heard referred to as the "third kidney"), lungs, kidney, and colon. Particularly helpful are B vitamins, folate, some of the amino acids, antioxidants, and many of the minerals.

A baby's organs of detoxification aren't fully developed at birth — a new baby can't sweat, the blood-brain barrier isn't fully developed, and the organs are still forming — and thus a newborn cannot detoxify adequately on their own.

You Are What You Eat 101

Every day, we need to consume **fats, protein, carbohydrates, vitamins, minerals, and water** to thrive. These nutrients are the building blocks of blood, bones, tissue, brain matter, and other organs. They also help detoxify the body.

- **Bones** are made up of protein and minerals.
- **Muscles** are made up of protein, vitamins, and minerals (including B12, iron, and folate).
- **The brain** is made up of fats and proteins.
- **The blood** is made up primarily of plasma (which is largely water, proteins, vitamins, and minerals) and red blood cells and a much smaller ration of white blood cells and platelets.
- **Organs** are made up of tissue, which is made up of cells.

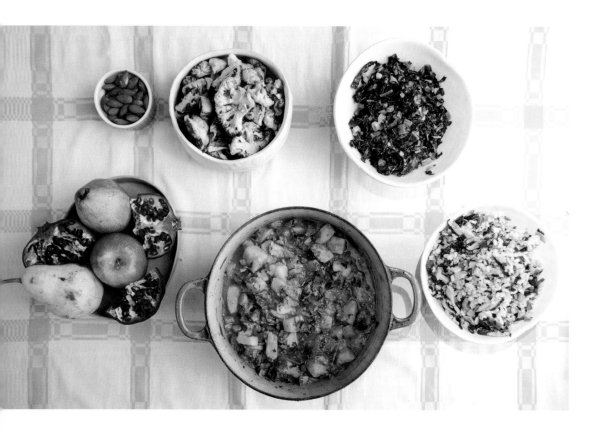

While we may continue to live if we aren't getting enough of some essential nutrients or trace minerals or vitamins, if we don't have enough of everything we need, the body starts stealing from itself, which it can only do for so long, and it can cause stress on the adrenal and thyroid glands, resulting in muscular soreness, brain fog, excessive fatigue, insomnia, hypoglycemia, and headaches. When a woman is pregnant, the baby takes its share of these elements, even if there isn't enough left over for the mother. If there isn't enough of, say, fat being ingested to build the baby's brain, the baby's brain will be affected.

Pregnancy and Cravings

If a woman goes into pregnancy with less-than-perfect digestion and nutrition, then she is likely to crave things — usually carbohydrates or sugars — that could destabilize her blood sugar or compromise her digestion. During pregnancy, cravings may be a sign of particular nutritional deficits. But it is unlikely your body needs ice cream, potato chips, or, in my case, hot and sour soup. If cravings were tied that directly to their corresponding nutrients, we would all crave kale, fish oil, and bone broth!

Even worse, sometimes the very foods we crave contain anti-nutrients, which stop our bodies from getting what they need out of the healthy foods we do eat. For example, while hot and sour soup may not seem an awful food to eat during pregnancy (and I ate a lot of it), it often contains a number of anti-nutrients, including MSG (which occurs in most soy sauce and is added to many Chinese dishes) and soy. MSG can block the body's absorption of taurine, which is essential in the development and functioning of the brain and nervous system and in the body's detoxification processes. Soy has been linked to other problems that I will discuss later.

An Introduction to Anti-Nutrients

Thanks to anti-nutrients, we can't eat crap and then dose up on the world's best vitamins. Anti-nutrients can be natural (such as isoflavones from soy or phytic acid from improperly prepared grains) or synthetic (food colouring, artificial sweeteners, or pesticides), and they can interfere with your body's ability to make use of the nutrients from the good food you do eat. Anti-nutrients can also harm your body's digestive process, lead to inflammation, and otherwise contribute to chronic conditions such as infertility, diabetes, obesity, osteoporosis, and Alzheimer's disease.

Some of the most troubling anti-nutrients are food additives, which can be natural or synthetic. Both can be problematic, especially for men and women concerned with their fertility or growing a child.

The Green Mama's List of the Seven Most Dangerous Food Additives

One of the most important first steps in healthy eating is to avoid food additives. All of the ingredients in the following list are considered safe by the Canadian and U.S. governments, but thanks to independent researchers, the data is piling up to prove they may be anything but safe.

1. **Artificial sweeteners, including aspartame (NutraSweet, Equal) and saccharin**
   Aspartame has been linked to the development of lymphomas, leukemia, and mammary cancer at levels "close to acceptable daily intake for humans," according to a study that also found increased carcinogenic effects if exposure began as a fetus. The FDA unsuccessfully set out to ban aspartame because of research suggesting it "might induce brain tumours." Studies have found that men who drink diet sodas are at increased risk for non-Hodgkin lymphomas and Type 2 diabetes.

2. **Artificial food colouring**
   Artificial food colouring was originally derived from coal tar (yes, the stuff used to patch roads) and is now more often derived from petroleum (as in what is used to fuel cars). They are often mixed with hydrocarbons like toluene, xylene, and benzene. All of these things are as bad as they sound: studies link their use with cancer in mice and hyperactivity in children. Some colours, such as Yellows 6 and 5, have been linked to endocrine disruption, which may contribute to breast cancer and lowered sperm counts. Researchers at the University of Southampton studied more than 1,800 children aged three years and found that, across the board, children behaved better without artificial food colourings and worse with them.

   You can learn more about spotting artificial food colouring in the **Label Reading 101** section later in this chapter. Thanks to a December 2016 law passed in Canada, food companies will now have to do more than just add the word *colour* to the label. (Not much more, but it's a start.)

3. **Carrageenan**
   This ingredient is used to thicken or stabilize certain foods, and it is found in many infant formulas, dairy alternatives, and all but one of my favourite brands of ice cream (*urgh*). It belongs to a family of molecules that can't be digested, but, because it comes from red algae, it's considered "natural." Small amounts in food are thought to be safe for adults, but the WHO has said it is inadvisable to use carrageenan in infant formula as it might be absorbed by the gut and affect the infant's developing immune system. A review of 45 available animal studies published in 2001 associated its use with the development of cancerous lesions in the colon.

4. **Fructose**

Wait, you are thinking, isn't fructose the better kind of sugar? Not so! Fructose triggers the body to make fat and blocks the ability of the body to burn fat. It depletes energy and triggers hunger. Liver cells break down fructose into a fat known as triglycerides. This also creates uric acid as waste. Both of these are linked with obesity, Type 2 diabetes, bad cholesterol, and fatty liver diseases. Studies suggest that a pregnancy diet high in fructose may harm the placenta, restrict fetal growth, and be associated with other pregnancy disorders such as preeclampsia and gestational diabetes. Fructose crosses the placenta so sugar addiction can start before kids are even born. Dr. Robert Lustig, author of *Fat Chance,* notes that the earlier you expose a child to sweets, the more they will crave it later. This includes exposure to infant formula, natural juices, and sweetened milks.

5. **Monosodium Glutamate (MSG)**

The main ingredient in MSG is free glutamic acid, or glutamate, which is considered "natural" because it is an amino acid. Naturally occurring glutamates aren't dangerous, but processed glutamates like MSG have been linked to short-term effects such as headaches, difficulty concentrating, skin reactions, mood swings, and depression. Some studies suggest it could play a part in neurodegenerative diseases such as Alzheimer's, Parkinson's, and Huntington's. For some people, MSG over-stimulates the nervous system, causing an inflammatory response that is cumulative in nature and so can get worse over time. Children and pregnant mothers in particular should avoid MSG because it can affect the developing fetus and alter the developing baby's brain.

MSG is the most prevalent of the food additives, so it's nearly impossible to totally avoid. A flavour enhancer, it works by over-exciting brain cell receptors. It can hide out under many different names, including autolyzed yeast, yeast extract, hydrolyzed proteins, sodium caseinate, calcium caseinate, plant protein extract, and soya sauce, and can even be found in some items with labels that state "natural flavourings," "does not contain MSG," and "organic."

6. **Nitrates**

When we digest foods that contain nitrates, our bodies form compounds called nitrosamines, which are known to be carcinogenic. Research suggests that mothers who eat nitrate-containing foods during pregnancy are more likely to have offspring who will develop brain tumours. The more nitrate-containing processed meats, the greater the risk to the child. Sodium nitrate/nitrites can be found in some food preservatives, lunch meats, bacon, pepperoni, hot dogs, and some well waters (usually near agricultural areas). Once again, because it can naturally occur in some vegetables, like celery, it's considered "natural." Thus, nitrates can still be found in meat products claiming to have all "natural ingredients" and "no added preservatives." The same research that found a connection between eating nitrate-containing processed meats and brain tumours found there was no such correlation with eating nitrate-containing vegetables. They also showed that women who took prenatal vitamins, especially with vitamins C and E, had less risk than those who did not.

7. **Trans Fats**

Fat is really important in our bodies. It works as a chemical messenger for our hormone systems, it repairs tissues, and it protects our organs. Our brain is 60 percent fat. Trans fats, masquerading as those oh-so-important healthy fats, displace essential fatty acids, but they can't do the job as well. The result is that they disrupt healthy fat balance and can harm the structure of the brain and nerve cells.

For babies-to-be, trans fats cross both the placenta to enter the blood of the fetus and, later, into breast milk. A pregnant or nursing mother's blood profile of trans fats will almost exactly match her baby's. In a pregnant mother, they are associated with low birth weights, smaller head circumference, problems in visual and central nervous system development, and preeclampsia. Dr. Jorge Chavarro, of the Harvard Nurse's study, found consuming trans fats increased the risk of infertility for both men and women.

Trans fatty acids (or "partially hydrogenated oils," as they often appear on labels) are found in things like margarine, vegetable shortening, fried restaurant foods, and microwave popcorn. Hydrogenated oils are made by first heating a vegetable oil to a high temperature, injecting it with a chemical solvent, and finishing it with bleach and a deodorizer.

"Natural" Anti-Nutrients

We might expect anti-nutrients when we eat a hot dog chased down with a diet float, but most people's biggest exposure to anti-nutrients comes from things they probably think are healthy. These include **cereal grains** (especially refined flour); **Omega-6 oils** from sources such as corn, cottonseed, safflower, and soybean oil; **sugar** and high-fructose corn syrup; and **processed soy** products such as soy milk, soy protein, and tofu.

Plants use anti-nutrients to protect themselves, so most plant-based food contains some anti-nutrients. Nutritionists have a "Top 10" list of naturally occurring anti-nutrients:

1. Phytic acid (found in grains and legumes)
2. Gluten (found in glutinous grains)

3. Flavonoids, such as tannins (tea, fruit skins, and wine)
4. Oxalates (soybeans, rhubarb, spinach, peanuts, chocolate)
5. Lectins (seeds, legumes, wheat, peanuts, soy)
6. Saponins (soy, chickpeas, and other beans)
7. Protease inhibitors, such as trypsin (soy, beans, grains, nuts, seeds, and night-shade vegetables, which include potatoes, tomatoes, eggplant, and peppers)
8. Isoflavones (soy)
9. Solanine (nightshade vegetables)
10. Amylase inhibitors (beans)

These natural anti-nutrients serve a function in moderation. Kale, wheat berry, and tomato plants need to have a little bit of protection to keep them from being eaten by all of the bugs. Ongoing research suggests that while eating too much of these naturally occurring anti-nutrients is likely bad, having a little bit might help balance blood sugar and protect us against cancer. The key is in preparation. Understanding how to properly prepare food will eliminate the negative effects of these natural anti-nutrients and leave the nutrition (and taste!) available to us. It's usually quite simple. Read more in the **How to Green Your Diet** section later in this chapter to learn why your grandmother soaked her beans and rice and babied her sourdough starter.

Essential Nutrients and Where to Find Them

The best sources of nutrients are from whole foods, because our bodies have evolved to access the most nutrients from whole sources. Procuring and preparing the most nutritious foods while minimizing anti-nutrients requires some vigilance when buying prepared food products, but it becomes easy when cooking simple ingredients from scratch. Even then, we may not get all the nutrients we need through our diets alone. Many foods are less nutritious than they were a hundred years ago because the soil they are grown in is more depleted of nutrients. (Just like we rely on nutrition to grow, plants rely on nutrients in soil.) In addition, there are far more toxins today than there ever were in the past, and these toxins can put undue stress on the body, further inhibiting our ability to access the nutrients that are in the food.

Consequently, most people need to supplement their diets for optimal health. Don't skimp. Poor-quality vitamins, like poor-quality food, will be lower in nutrients and higher in anti-nutrients. Look for a prenatal vitamin that is made from real, organic food without added dyes, artificial flavours, or fillers. Pay particular attention to getting essential fatty acids from fish oil (which will include vitamin A), vitamin D, vitamin K, magnesium, folate (not folic acid), iodine, and iron (if you need it), and consider supplementing with a high-quality probiotic.

Fats

Fats are essential to our health. They help to build your growing baby's brain and eyes. They surround the cells of your body and build the hormones that underlie a healthy pregnancy. You and your baby's nervous systems contain more DHA (from omega-3 fats) than any other tissue, and you need a lot of DHA and EPA (also from omega-3 fats) for the nervous system to function well. During pregnancy, the fetus takes from the mother all the fats she needs to develop her brain and nervous system. This exchange continues through the breastfeeding relationship. In order for the baby to get the nutrients he needs for optimal brain, visual, and neurological development — and for a mother's brain to function well — they both need the right kinds of fats before, during, and after pregnancy. These include the **essential fats** (aka essential fatty acids), such as the aforementioned omega-3. These are necessary for life but aren't made by the body and so must be supplied through food.

Besides omega-3, omega-6 essential fatty acid is the other big player in the functioning of the body and brain. Unfortunately, the optimal ratio between these fats is way out of whack in most humans, and this imbalance is causing health issues. We used to eat diets that were nearly balanced in omega-3 and omega-6. Today, however, our diets give us approximately 16 times more omega-6 than omega-3. This excess of omega-6s in the diet can cause chronic inflammation and be a factor in the development of many common diseases, including allergies, asthma, cardiovascular disease, Type 2 diabetes, and joint pain.

It's not that omega-6 fatty acids are bad. Inflammation is the body's appropriate response to injury. The problem is a lopsided ratio that can lead to chronic inflammation and the diseases that go with it. The solution is to eat less omega-6 and more omega-3. The primary sources of omega-6 in most North American diets are processed seed and vegetable oils such as sunflower, corn, soy, cottonseed, and canola (in roughly that order). The biggest contributor in most diets is soy oil, namely because it can be cheaply produced, making it a popular ingredient in many processed foods. Start looking for this ingredient on labels and you will see why omega-6 stores have increased so dramatically in human fat and breast milk.

The richest sources of omega-3s, which include all-important DHA and EPA, are marine sources such as seafood and fish oil. There are plant-based sources, *sort of*. Flaxseed, pumpkin seed, walnut oils, and seaweed all contain a precursor nutrient that must then be turned into EPA and DHA to be useful. The problem is that most bodies aren't very efficient at this conversion. It's hard to get enough of the most necessary essential fats without relying upon animal sources. Yet researchers suggest that most of us will benefit from more of all the sources of omega-3, so don't stop eating those plant-based sources as well!

Seafood is the best source. Studies show that women who consume fish or fish oil have smarter children than those who do not, even though studies also show that neurotoxins accumulate in fish, especially the neurotoxin mercury, which can cause severe developmental issues in children. To put it really simply: fish contain omega-3s, which make your kids smart, and they also contain mercury, which can make them dumb. The longer-living, and often bigger fish, tend to have more mercury, and more mercury makes kids less smart. So, what is a mother-to-be to do?

I recommend you still eat fish, just eat safer fish. And take a daily dose of supplemental cod liver or fish oil that has been tested and certified mercury-free (read up on the added benefit of fermented cod liver oil). It's recommended that pregnant women eat the equivalent of two servings of fatty fish a week or take the equivalent of 200 mg of DHA from fish oil supplements. Most women today get far less than this. It is also important to supplement your diet with DHA long after pregnancy and breastfeeding to replenish your body's stores. Doing so can even help protect against postpartum depression. Read **Baby- and Mama-Safe Seafood** on page 46 to learn which fresh seafood is best for you, your baby-to-be, and the fish populations.

Animal products can also be rich sources of omega-3 as long as they are exposed to sunlight and pasture or grass and are raised using organic techniques. Animals raised in such a manner have fat stores with more omega-3 and less omega-6 than conventional sources. The best omega-3 animal sources are eggs, particularly the yolk, from pastured chickens and the organs and meat from ruminants fed grass — that includes beef, bison, lamb, and goat. Pork and chicken have less of many of the essential nutrients, including omega-3 fats, and more omega-6, but as long as they are raised along the lines of organic standards and allowed to eat grass and other natural feeds, rather than a diet based on grains, they will also be a decent source of some omega-3. A recent Canadian study found that the omega-3 to omega-6 ratio in butters was particularly bad in Canada, where our butter has become more like the ratio of those to-be-shunned vegetable oils above. The culprit? Our industrial feeding practices and all the soy and corn in dairy cows' diets. The good news is that organic butter from grass-fed cows can be sourced from farmers' markets or at certain grocery and specialty stores in Canada.

Plant-based sources of omega-3 include walnuts, chia seeds, flax seeds, sea vegetables, natto (a traditional Japanese food made from soybeans), Brussels sprouts, kale, spinach, and watercress.

The best oils for cooking and eating include ghee (clarified butter), extra-virgin olive oil, avocado oil, macadamia oil, duck fat, lard from organic and pastured animals, walnut oil, unsalted grass-fed butter (not good for high-temperature cooking), and flax oil (but not good with even medium-high heat).

Synthetic omega-3 supplementation is best avoided. There is a growing trend to add omega-3 supplementation to foods ranging from conventionally raised dairy to juice boxes and baby food. The problem is that most omega-3 supplements taste fishy, so these foods must then undergo processes to remove the flavour. In my opinion, there isn't enough research to suggest that the end result is actually safe and effective.

Baby- and Mama-Safe Seafood

Fish and seafood can be great for growing brains, preventing depression, and general health. Unfortunately, seafood can also contain mercury and PCBs (polychlorinated biphenyl). Despite these contaminants, research indicates that women who eat fish during pregnancy have smarter children. So don't avoid seafood and fish; just eat it wisely.

The **healthiest and safest choices** for seafood and fish for Mama, Papa, Baby, and the Earth are

- Anchovies
- Farmed Arctic char
- Farmed oysters
- Farmed rainbow trout
- Wild Atlantic mackerel
- Wild sardines
- Wild Alaskan salmon (chum, coho, or sockeye)

Enzymes and Their Helpers

It's not just the fats; enzymes and coenzymes also keep things in the right balance. They play a major role in taking away both natural and synthetic toxins in the body. Dietary factors, such as anti-nutrients, can really mess things up in the enzyme world. Vitamin A and the B vitamins, including B2 (riboflavin), B3 (niacin), B5, and B6, as well as vitamins C and E and magnesium and zinc are necessary precursors to enzymes.

Folate is perhaps one of the best known of the enzyme helpers. It is essential for women before and during pregnancy. Folate promotes healthy neural tube formation, adequate birth weight, and proper development of the fetus's face and heart. Folate, which naturally occurs in foods such as liver and lentils, should not be confused with folic acid, which is not normally found in foods. Folic acid can be converted into usable forms of folate, but that conversion is limited. Also, folic acid does not cross the placenta like natural folate. Consuming too much folic acid from supplements — even at the recommended 400 mcg per day — can lead to high levels of un-metabolized folic acid in the blood, which can mask B12 deficiency, depress immune function, and even promote the development of certain cancers.

This does not lessen the importance of folate for mothers-to-be. Nutritionist Margaret Floyd Barry recommends a total of 800 mcg to 900 mcg per day. Ideally we would meet the need through food, but that is difficult for most women to accomplish. Remember, a nutrient eaten is *not* the same as a nutrient absorbed. Folate absorption in particular relies on having enough zinc in the body. To get enough zinc *and* folate, most women will need to increase their food sources (such as really high-quality organic liver, properly prepared legumes, and lots of dark leafy greens) *and* take a supplement. Since most supplements use folic acid instead of folate (it's easier and cheaper), seek out a special folate supplement from your local health food store or on the internet. Look on the ingredient list and *avoid* anything that says folic acid on the list, and instead *choose* something with folate, 5-methyl-tetrahydrofolate, L-methylfolate, or Metfolin.

Choline is related to the all-important folate and has an even more direct role in the development of a child's brain and nervous system. It provides protection against neurotoxins. The RDA (recommended daily allowance) for pregnant women is 450 mg per day, but more can be beneficial and will not be harmful. Choline can be obtained from organic, grass-fed organ meats such as liver, kidneys, and brain, as well as egg yolk, whole dairy, caviar, fish roe and some fish, nuts, legumes, and cruciferous vegetables (broccoli, cabbage, cauliflower, kale, collards, turnip, Chinese cabbage, and radish, for example).

Vitamin A plays an integral role in developing the cells, tissues, and organs within the body, including the brain. The current RDA of vitamin A for pregnant women is 2,600 IU, but keepers of traditional wisdom say it should be much higher, ideally 20,000 IU and preferably from cod liver oil. Vitamin A is found

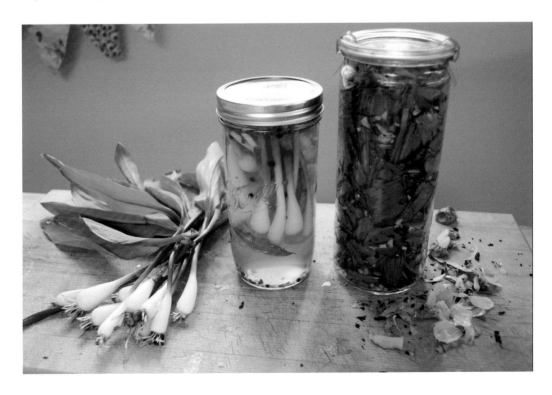

in high-quality, organic organ meats (especially liver); whole milk, butter, and eggs; and in the aforementioned cod liver oil (but make sure you get one with naturally occurring amounts rather than synthetic vitamin A).

Vitamin K, or potassium, is best known for helping the blood to clot. We are just beginning to fully understand all of its other benefits, one of which is to work with vitamin D to help with overall health. Vitamin K keeps calcium in the bones and out of soft tissue, and deficiency of it is thought to play a part in varicose veins, osteoporosis, tooth decay, brain problems, and a number of cancers. It is a fat-soluble vitamin that we can't make ourselves and doesn't store well; thus, many people are deficient in vitamin K, especially K2, which works in the blood vessels and bones. Vitamin K1 is found in leafy greens, while vitamin K2 is found in fermented foods, grass-fed animal fats, and the naturally fermented Japanese soybean called natto, as well as in goose liver, cheese, egg yolks, and butter.

Vitamin D helps build bones and develop the lungs of the growing baby. These days vitamin D is considered a sort of wonder vitamin that also helps with weight management, mood, and overall health. One study specifically looking at vitamin D and pregnancy found that women who took 4,000 IU of vitamin D every day in their second and third trimesters showed no evidence of harm but had half the rate of pregnancy complications (such as gestational diabetes, preterm birth, and preeclampsia) as those that took only the recommended 400 IU. Vitamin D comes from sunlight and fats from animals "fed" sunlight, either because they were allowed to graze outside or, for seafood, ate a lot of plankton or seaweed. It's nearly impossible to get enough vitamin D from the sun, particularly in Canada. Unless you eat a lot of cod liver oil, fatty fish, and lard, you probably don't get enough from your diet alone either. (African-American women were the most likely to be deficient in vitamin D, followed by Hispanic women. The darker one's skin, the more vitamin D that may be required.) Mothers who are deficient are more likely to have babies that are deficient in vitamin D, and this continues through the breastfeeding relationship.

Magnesium deficiency is one of the leading nutrient deficiencies. It affects an estimated 80 percent of people. The body uses magnesium in everyday activities such as the heart beating, production of hormones, muscle movement, and metabolism. Although we only need relatively small amounts of magnesium, this nutrient must be replenished constantly, either from food or supplementation, in order to keep deficiencies from developing. Magnesium levels are affected by too little or too much calcium, vitamin K, and vitamin D.

Magnesium can be found in dark leafy greens, nuts and seeds, fish, beans and lentils, whole grains, and bone broth. Because of soil depletion, it can be hard to get enough through your food. It can, however, be supplemented through the skin in a spray-on supplement. Its use may even help with symptoms of nausea in pregnancy. Pregnant women need 350 mg to 360 mg of magnesium daily.

Vitamin E was called Fertility Factor X after it was discovered that rats could not reproduce without it, and then it was renamed *tocopherol*, from the Greek "to bring forth childbirth." Vitamin E is thought to be essential in building the nutritional transport system of the human placenta. It can be found in palm oil, animal fats, nuts, seeds, fresh fruits and vegetables, and freshly ground grains.

Iron deficiency or anemia is very common in pregnancy and should be checked for in your routine blood work. If you are low in iron, eating foods rich in heme iron will ensure the iron is more easily absorbed and be less likely to cause constipation. These sources include liver, beef, clams, and oysters. Plant foods are a source of non-heme iron. Heme iron is typically absorbed at a rate of 7 to 35 percent; non-heme iron is typically absorbed at a rate of 2 to 20 percent. If your maternity care provider also recommends an iron supplement, it is advised that you take it apart from the rest of your vitamins because other vitamins can interfere with its absorption. Iron chelate is supposedly the most non-constipating form in supplements. Taking vitamin C (in supplement form or in vitamin C–rich foods) makes the iron more absorbable; calcium (such as from your leafy greens or milk or from a supplement) blocks absorption.

How to Green Your Diet to Grow a Happy, Healthy Baby

Here are a series of action steps listed from ♥♥♥ (biggest impact, and possibly more work) to ♥ (quick and easy) to help you green your womb for your child and for future generations.

1. ♥♥♥ **Organic-ize your diet.** Know what foods to eat beyond organic (for example, grass-fed meats and dairy), what foods to always buy organic (for example, your leafy greens), and which foods you can cheat on and when. Read the **Organic-ize Your Diet** section for guidance, but when in doubt, buy and eat certified organic, as it's a trustworthy label that will protect you and your baby-to-be from food additives and residue from chemical pesticides. It may even help you get more nutrition per bite.

2. ♥♥♥ **Focus on your digestive health.** Read your poop for clues: if it floats or has undigested food in it, is very firm or very loose, or is less frequent than once a day, you probably need digestive support. Try the tips in this chapter to help improve your digestion. If this doesn't work, consider working with a functional nutritionist. Betaine hydrochloride, which supports the production of hydrochloric acid in your stomach, may help. Margaret Floyd Barry says it may be the single most important supplement a person

can take. Getting help to support your digestion is one of the best investments you can make. Your baby is depending on every bit she can get for growing a strong body and big brain.

3. ♥♥♥ **Learn to prepare your food in a healthier way.** Yes, even really healthy foods, like all those leafy greens and organic legumes that are so essential to the health of your growing baby, should be prepared to minimize their naturally occurring anti-nutrients. In short:

- **Rinse.** Rinse all of your foods, even the organic ones, to remove dirt, germs, and any pesticide residue. When rinsing grains or legumes, rinse until the water runs clear.
- **Soak.** Soaking, especially your legumes and grains, helps remove a significant portion of the anti-nutrients. I recommend soaking most legumes and grains at least overnight, but most beans do well with an even longer soak. Some of these will release a soapy or scummy film that should be disposed of before and during cooking. It can help to use a tablespoon of whey, yogourt, or lemon when soaking to further break down the anti-nutrients and to help release the enzyme phytase, which will further break down phytic acid and release other beneficial nutrients. For instance, put your oatmeal or porridge in the pot the night before with warm water and a bit of yogourt, and let it soak overnight. (To learn about how to properly prepare grains, I particularly recommend the book *Nourishing Traditions* by Sally Fallon Morell.)
- **Sprout.** Sprouting is a great way to break down anti-nutrients and make the nutrients more digestible. Most seeds (except chia and flax) can be sprouted, but don't eat alfalfa sprouts, which are particularly high in a number of anti-nutrients, including L-cavanine and saponins, and can also be contaminated by salmonella and E. coli. See the **Green Eating Recipe Handbook** on pages 64–71 to learn how to soak-sprout your own nuts.
- **Ferment.** Fermenting grains as a sourdough can break down anti-nutrients, such as gluten, and it tastes great. You can capture your own sourdough, or you can buy a sourdough starter on the internet or at your local natural food store.

    Fermenting vegetables is a really easy way to start fermenting. It breaks down anti-nutrients in raw foods and introduces healthy bacteria into your gut. A food that you ferment yourself can be way more effective at this than even a probiotic supplement. You can start as easily as making your own sauerkraut or nonalcoholic ginger "beer" or ale. See the **Green Eating Recipe Handbook** on pages 64–71 to get started. From these you can move on to fermenting other vegetables, making flavourful kimchi, or trying other drinks such as kefir or tibicos. I highly recommend Sandor Katz's book *Wild Fermentation* for additional recipes.

4. ♥♥♥ **Adopt a diet rich in nutrients.** This will involve eating regular servings of mama-safe seafood, coconut oil, organic and grass-fed butter and liver, real milk, beef and other fatty animal proteins, eggs, bone broth, lots of all sorts of vegetables (especially leafy greens), fermented foods and beverages, whole fruits, and properly prepared grains.

5. ♥♥ **Eat home-cooked meals.** In North America we are in a weird food bubble where food is cheaper than anywhere else relative to spending, and we spend way more of our food budget out in restaurants than our peers around the world do. It's very unlikely that you can get someone else to prepare food with ingredients as high quality as you would at home for the same money. Save your food dollars for better food, and prepare and eat more meals at home.

6. ♥♥ **Learn to make bone broth.** Bone broth from high-quality meat sources is one of the most cost-effective mineral- and nutrient-rich foods that a person can eat. It is right up there with fish oil, egg yolks, real milk, and grass-fed butter in its importance in a pregnancy and postpartum diet. Bone broth, aka stock, contains minerals in a form easily digestible. While it is not the food with the highest amounts of calcium, magnesium, phosphorous, silicon, or sulfur, it does have them and numerous other nutrients in one of the most easily absorbable forms. As well, bone broth is rich in gelatin, which can help ease food sensitivities and gut imbalances. That gelatin comes from the breakdown of collagen in the animal bones. Collagen is the most abundant protein in the human body. It builds healthy bones, cartilage, skin, arteries, and the placenta. To get started making your own homemade broth, see the **Green Eating Recipe Handbook**.

7. ♥♥ **Learn to read labels** in order to avoid the worst food additives and other anti-nutrients. Remember that with many food additives, the chemicals of concern are considered natural and thus can hide under inconspicuous titles such as *natural flavouring*. The best-researched foodies these days say that if your great-grandmother (or someone's great-grandmother) wasn't eating it, then it's probably not real food. In other words, your great-grandma wasn't eating that strange no-fat yogourt in a squeeze pouch or that can of soup or that vitamin water, so you'd be better off without it, too.

8. ♥♥ **Eat the most important foods — that's the fat, protein, and vegetables — first, and then finish with the starches.** Do that for each meal and throughout the day in general. You will find your blood sugar and mood will thank you.

A Better Cuppa

Tea

I start every morning with a cup of tea. This is because black, green, white, and all the variations of tea are full of antioxidant-rich flavonoids. Well, actually, maybe it's just because I love the taste and ritual, and coffee makes me loopy. Unfortunately, tea leaves can contain a *lot* of pesticide residue. And some of the most popular brands are some of the most contaminated. These include Celestial Seasonings, Tetley, Bigelow, Twinings, Mighty Leaf, Teavanna, Republic of Tea, Yogi, Tea Forte, Trader Joe's, Tazo, and David's Teas, according to a study by Eurofins. Many of these teas far exceed what's considered safe levels of pesticide exposure. Since those standards are pretty questionable to begin with, that's a big cup of pesticides. Yuck! Even worse, these teas disguise other known or suspected toxins, such as artificial food colourings, under the term "natural flavourings."

Tea is made from the leaves, and sometimes stems, of the Camellia sinensis plant and is often grown in China or India. The pesticides used on these plants have very little chance for removal before becoming part of our morning routine. Luckily, drinking organic loose-leaf tea will significantly reduce exposure to pesticides, while maximizing the health benefits of good-quality tea.

Coffee

North Americans drink a lot of coffee. Research suggests that coffee can also have antioxidant health benefits, but drinkers — and especially workers — can suffer from the intensive pesticides used in production. Look for certified organic coffee — shade-grown isn't the same — to ensure you and the farm workers are both looked after.

Buying organic tea and coffee is especially important when buying decaf. That's because most coffee and tea is decaffeinated using chemicals, including the possibly carcinogenic chemical methyl chloride (dichloromethane) and the slightly less toxic ethyl acetate, of which traces can be left behind. More natural methods of decaffeination include using carbon dioxide or just water and osmosis, known as the Swiss Water process (developed in Burnaby, British Columbia, by the way!). Only the carbon dioxide or Swiss Water methods are allowed in coffees certified organic.

9. ♥♥ **Filter your water.** Tap water and bottled water, even in North America, can be sources of parasites and bacteria as well as other contaminants. A lot of tap water also contains lead from old pipes. Similarly, some scientists believe that our overexposure to fluoride — found in much of North America's drinking water — is lowering IQ, weakening bones, and delaying the eruption of teeth. Don't take this information and go running toward the arms of the bottled water industry. Bottled water has even fewer regulations protecting it and devastates the environment using 1.5 million barrels of oil a year. Buying bottled water would cost a family of four over $1,200 a year. Instead, I suggest you invest in a good water filtration system for your home and carry either a glass or stainless steel bottle for drinking. You can buy a countertop product, such as a Berkey. It rarely requires new filters and is less than $400, but it is slow. The under-the-counter options filter much faster but usually are more expensive, and they need their filters replaced more often. You will pay extra to remove the fluoride, but preliminary research suggests that it's worth it. If you don't have access to a water filter or truly cannot afford one, you can lower the lead content in water (that might come from old pipes) by letting the water run at the tap for at least ten seconds before filling your cup or pot.

10. ♥♥ **Reduce the amount of plastics in your kitchen and your diet.** This includes from food packaging: cans, food taken out from restaurants put into Styrofoam, plastic, or non-stick paper. It is safer and more environmentally conscious to use ceramic, glass, or stainless steel containers, which come with few safety concerns and are more easily reused. Learn more about the toxins in plastics in the **Green Mama-to-Be*ware*** appendix at the end of the book.

11. ♥♥ **Make sure your coffee or tea is organic and naturally decaffeinated.** The pesticide residue from the growing process and the chemicals used in most decaffeination processes include many known toxins. Some of the most popular brands are the worst offenders. You can protect yourself by buying certified organic teas and coffee, which means that they are grown without toxic pesticides and that if they are decaffeinated, the process is done without dangerous chemicals. I've always found it hard to find my favourite loose-leaf tea certified organic and decaffeinated, so I buy the organic and decaffeinate it myself. Decaffeinated doesn't mean without caffeine: decaf tea or coffee can have 1 to 20 percent of the original caffeine. To decaffeinate your own loose-leaf tea at home, all you have to do is steep your tea leaves in hot water for 30 seconds to one minute, then drain this first rinse off and re-steep. It is estimated that almost 70 percent of the caffeine is removed in the first brew.

12. ♥ **Don't routinely drink juice, soda, sport drinks, or fancy coffee drinks.** Drinks, even the kinds without added sugar, pack a powerful punch on blood sugar. Without the added fibre to slow down absorption, they not only mess with blood sugar, but they also make it hard to absorb any supposed nutrients. This makes their calories empty. Even worse, the over-consumption of sugar can program the unborn child toward a sugar addiction.

13. ♥ **Take a food-based organic prenatal supplement.** Make sure the supplement has folate (not folic acid). Also consider supplementing with high-quality fish oil, such as cod liver (without synthetic additives); additional vitamin D; vitamin K; magnesium; and a high-quality probiotic.

14. ♥ **Eat a variety of flavours.** Your baby can taste what you eat through the amniotic fluid, which can be flavoured by your food choices. You can set the foundation of your future child's diverse food tastes by eating sour, spicy, and bitter flavours as well as the usual sweet and savoury.

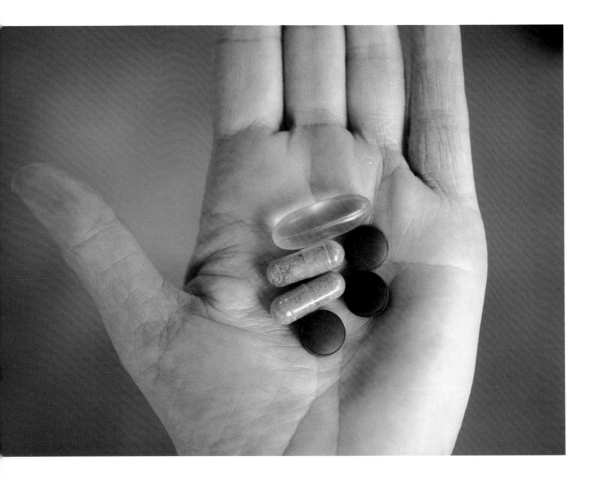

Organic-ize Your Diet

Organic Eating 101: It's Important

Every functional nutritionist, toxin scientist, and holistic medical professional that I spoke with for this book and the first *Green Mama* book says that children and parents-to-be, especially moms while pregnant, should prioritize eating organic. The evidence is all too clear: pesticides in foods have been linked by many credible scientific studies and extensive research to obesity, autism, cancer, birth defects, and neurological problems in children.

The good news is that we can limit our own and our children's exposure to many of the worst toxins by eating organic. Studies have shown that children who eat primarily organic produce have fewer pesticides in their bodies than their conventional eating counterparts. Eating organic is an effective strategy for lowering exposure to antibiotics and artificial growth hormones, as well. Organic foods can also be more nutritious per bite and especially high in antioxidants.

If you occasionally feel conflicted about organics, I can relate. On the one hand, reading the studies and speaking to the experts makes me believe in the importance of organic. But many people can't afford to eat organic, including my own family members, such as my sister, who just had her third child. Luckily, the price differential on organics has gotten slimmer and continues to decrease with the prevalence of organic sections in most grocery stores and the increase in farmers' markets.

Organic foods are a multi-billion-dollar industry that is growing fast. The majority of Canadians — that's 20 million people — say they regularly buy organics.

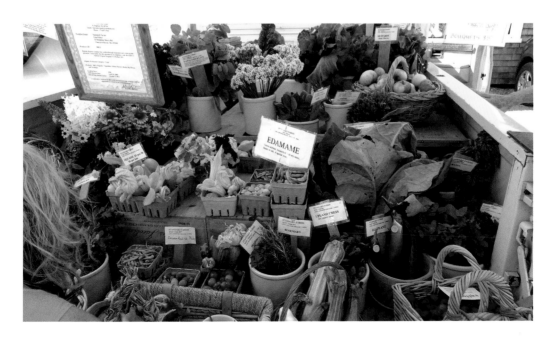

Eighty-six percent of Canadians, particularly those in the 18- to 36-year-old demographic, say they expect to continue or increase their organic spending.

I believe the most important foods to buy organic are dairy and meat (including poultry), though this accounts for less than a quarter of Canadian organic purchases.

Organic Shopping 101: Where to Spend Your Food Dollars

The keys to organic-izing your diet are to know how to best spend your food dollars by understanding when it is important to buy organic, when organic isn't enough, and where you can save your money and go for conventional instead. An important tool is learning to read labels so that you don't accidentally get fooled into spending more for something unless it truly is better.

1. **Go beyond organic for animal products.** The most important foods to eat beyond organic (organic *and* pasture-raised) are animal products. This includes meat, poultry, dairy, and eggs. Making sure you go beyond organic to find animals fed their natural diets and given access to sunlight means you will get more nutrients, as well. Remember the Canadian cows with their poor-quality butter? The solution is to find organic butter from grass-fed livestock. Similarly, chickens raised in pastures with real sunlight lay eggs that contain more vitamin A and beta carotene, omega-3 fatty acids, vitamin E, and vitamin D than eggs collected from chickens living in indoor cages. Organic isn't enough when buying fish either. Learn more about this and how to find better animal products in the **Label Reading 101** section.

2. **Keep in mind that natural isn't the same as organic.** Natural isn't a meaningful, third-party certified label. It can mean just about anything. This can be especially tricky for processed meat products, such as hot dogs, salami, lunch meats, and bacon, all of which can contain high levels of nitrates and still be labelled "all natural." I enjoy the taste and convenience of processed meat products, but their consumption has been linked to certain cancers. I recommend you buy these products organic and frozen, without preservatives. Better yet, make your own by cutting thin slices of home-roasted chicken breast or beef and freezing it.

3. **Buy organic oils.** Cooking oils, even those from vegetables, can contain pesticides. Similarly, you want oils to be minimally refined to get the most from their nutrients, such as certified organic virgin olive oil.

4. **Buy organic grains.** This includes breads, pastas, and other grain products. Grains are a relatively pesticide-intensive crop. When grains are packaged into a food, you can't rinse them to remove any chemical residue.

5. **Rice.** Even organic rice can have very high levels of arsenic from contaminated groundwater in many rice-growing areas. Women and children are

advised to limit their rice consumption to once a week and to properly rinse and soak rice to help minimize exposure. I love rice and eat it regularly; I minimize exposure by limiting all forms of processed rice, such as rice crackers and breads, and saving my exposure for eating rice dishes. I also buy organic rice from more mountainous areas, where the groundwater is cleaner, and I often mix my brown rice with (generally less contaminated) white rice. Rinsing and soaking rice before use can also help. So can cooking it with excess water and then refreshing it after it first boils.

6. **Make sure you buy organic baby food (or anything else that is concentrated).** If you eat a lot of something, whatever that is, make sure it's organic. And if you are eating a lot of something concentrated like ketchup, make sure it's organic. This is because in concentrated foods like baby food and ketchup, any pesticides in the ingredients could be concentrated as well. Remember, too, that a baby eats more per pound and drinks more by volume than an adult. And his developing system is far more vulnerable to pesticides.

7. **Know the most important fruits and veggies to buy organic.** The Environmental Working Group refers to the most contaminated fruits and veggies as "The Dirty Dozen" and looks at the average amount of pesticide residue on commonly eaten fruits and vegetables (after it is washed or peeled). Conventional apples can contain the residue of 42 different pesticides, and conventional celery 64. Yikes. (If you want to check out a particular food, you can scare yourself silly at the website www.whatson myfood.org). To avoid the most pesticides on your fruits and veggies, here are the ones I would strongly suggest you always buy organic:

- Peaches/nectarines/apples/pears/plums (and other orchard fruits)
- Celery
- Berries, including strawberries, blueberries, cherries, and red raspberries
- Tomatoes
- Sweet bell peppers and hot peppers
- Leafy greens, including spinach, kale, collard greens, and lettuce
- Potatoes
- Grapes (especially those that are imported)
- Carrots
- Summer squash and zucchini
- Cucumbers
- Hawaiian pineapples

Less contaminated fruits and vegetables include onions, avocados, asparagus, frozen sweet peas, mangos, kiwis, domestic cantaloupes, and sweet potatoes.

Label Reading 101: What's Behind the Label

Organic/Biologique

To be able to use the word *organic* on a food label in Canada or the U.S., the product must have at least 70 percent organic ingredients and be free of GMOs and the worst of the food additives. A **Certified Organic** product contains at least 95 percent organic ingredients, and has an official USDA or Canada Organic/Biologique label. These products are grown without chemical herbicides, pesticides, fungicides, fertilizers, sewage sludge, or GMOs. Animals raised organically have access to pasture, eat organic feed that contains no antibiotics, and do not receive synthetic growth hormones. Organic products cannot be irradiated or have synthetic additives. The USDA Organic label can also be used on personal care products that meet the organic food standard for their products, meaning they are not only organic but made of edible ingredients. Canada does not have a similar option.

Canada's organic label has come under criticism recently because, unlike in the United States, Canada does not require field tests and it outsources certification in countries such as China that have questionable environmental standards. Nonetheless, the Certified Organic label for food is still the best assurance of quality.

Cage-Free, Free-Range, Grass-Fed, Hormone-Free, Antibiotic-Free, Natural, or All-Natural

These terms can be used without the independent verification that a third party provides. This makes them meaningless. Add to the list "No Antibiotics Used" or "No additional hormones added." When I see one of these terms without a third-party certification, I assume the company is greenwashing. Here's who certifies.

Meat/Poultry

The **Animal Welfare Approved** (AWA) label certifies small, independent farms that give their animals access to grass pasture, don't use growth hormones, don't routinely use antibiotics, and provide humane slaughtering practices. **Certified Humane** is a similar, less rigorous standard. It is available to corporate farms and doesn't require that the animals have had access to the outdoors. The **grass-fed label**, certified by the Food Alliance, the American Grassfed Association, or the USDA, requires that animals eat a grass diet although they may still have been confined to pens or feedlots. The Global Animal Partnership **5-Step Animal Welfare Rating**, developed by Whole Foods and now with third-party certification, offers a range of options. A "5+" represents the highest quality of organic animal husbandry but all steps prohibit growth hormones and the routine use of antibiotics.

Unfortunately, kosher and halal labels do not restrict growth hormones, pesticide residue, or antibiotic use. Similarly, "natural" means something has been minimally processed, but it does not restrict artificial growth hormones, antibiotic use, or pesticide residues.

Eggs

For the best eggs, look for labels such as **AWA**, or certified by the **Canadian Organic Regime**, the **Certified Organic Association of BC**, **Pro-Cert**, or **BC SPCA**. These labels indicate that the hens aren't fed antibiotics and spend time running around outdoors, rather than being locked inside overcrowded barns (with the exception of those labelled "Free-Run," which means they are given area to run around only indoors).

Eggs labelled "vegetarian fed" is almost a certain indicator that the chicken has been raised entirely indoors and fed grain. This isn't a healthy diet for chickens and consequently doesn't make the healthiest eggs for human consumption either.

The best options for eggs are those that are certified organic and pastured with one or more of the above labels to back it up. Or find a neighbour or farmer near you who raises their own hens in their backyard and see for yourself if they are given access to pasture and organic feed.

Fair Trade

FLO-CERT and **Fair to Life** are two organizations that certify products or ingredients to ensure that farmers are paid a living wage and are treated fairly. They support co-operatives and family farms, especially in the developing world, and minimize middle men. Their growers use sustainable farming practices with limited agrochemicals and no GMOs. This can be a particularly meaningful label when buying products, such as textiles or coffee, where there are often particularly unfair labour practices.

Sustainable Seafood

The USDA and Canada Organic/Biologique labels are currently meaningless when it comes to fish, so be wary when you see seafood labelled as organic. Proposed standards are on the way. In the meantime, other labels exist to indicate you are getting fish that was caught with respect to the health of the oceans, was not cloned or fed GMO food, and wasn't treated with the heavy doses of antibiotics fed to most farm-raised fish.

In general, seafood labels focus on the health of fishery stocks. The **Marine Stewardship Council** label indicates that seafood is wild-caught and the fishery is practising some care of fish stocks. **Seafood Watch** by the Monterey Bay Aquarium provides guides for sustainable fisheries by region. Canadians have a similar system called **SeaChoice** and the Vancouver Aquarium's **Ocean Wise** certification. Greenpeace posts a Red List of the most endangered food fish species on its website.

To find seafood that is lower in mercury and other contaminants, Seafood Watch maintains a **Super Green List** and the **KidSafeSeafood** program reports seafood choices that are gentler on both Earth and body. Read the **Mama & Baby Safe Seafood** box on page 46 to learn about the best seafood to eat and more about how to find truly wild salmon.

Salmon

Living on the West Coast of Canada, I have learned a lot about salmon. The most important take-away of which is to never eat farmed salmon. Farmed salmon is routinely contaminated with antibiotics and food dye, and in Canada and the U.S. it might be genetically engineered (aka cloned). It also tends to have "significantly higher" levels of organo-chlorine contaminants such as PCBs and PBDEs (polybrominated diphenyl ether), according to a 2004 study in the *American Journal of Environmental Science and Technology*.

How Do I Avoid Eating Farmed Salmon?
Unfortunately, Canada has weaker labelling regulations than either Europe or the United States. Fish in Canada can be sold without labelling to reveal anything about it, such as whether it is farmed, if it contains artificial dyes, or if it is genetically engineered. So you need to be aware. It is possible to find truly wild salmon by following these tips:

1. **Beware of the labels "Atlantic salmon" or "Wild Atlantic salmon,"** because it is farmed. There are no truly wild Atlantic salmon fisheries in Canada because the Atlantic salmon is an endangered species. Most of Canada's Atlantic salmon is farmed in the Pacific, so it's not even Atlantic in origin, just in breed.
2. **Only buy wild Pacific salmon.** Of course, the ideal is to find a local fisherman selling his wares from his boat or at your local farmers' market. Since that isn't an option for most people, you can buy from a fish vendor who takes pride in knowing his sources. Also, look for labels to back up environmental claims, such as those by the Marine Stewardship Council. Learn more about reading labels for fish, and all products, in the **Label Reading 101** section.

NON-GMO or GMO-Free

GMOs — or genetically modified organisms — aka GM or GE (genetically engineered) refer to plants or animals created through the changing or merging of a species' DNA. Canada allows GM varieties of corn, soy, sugar beets, canola, apples, and salmon. It's the fourth largest producer of GM crops, well behind the U.S. and Brazil. We also import GM cottonseed oil, papaya, and squash. rGBH tainted milk products come from the U.S. in processed foods that contain milk solids or powders such as frozen desserts or mixed drinks with dairy. In the 20 years since GM ingredients were first introduced into Canada, these foods have made their way into most of the processed foods available in Canada. Unless you buy foods labelled organic or NON-GMO, you are almost certainly getting them in packaged foods that contain corn, canola, soy, or sugar.

Unless the GMO-free claim is backed up with the NON-GMO Project label or, even better, one of the Certified Organic labels mentioned above, it's a meaningless claim. It should be noted that the NON-GMO label does not mean that a product is organic. Indeed, having a NON-GMO label on something like strawberries is meaningless as strawberries are not currently being genetically modified anywhere, yet they are a pesticide-intensive crop. You are far better-off spending the money on the organic strawberries or skipping over all the conventional strawberries, including the NON-GMO ones.

Gluten-Free and Other Allergen Labelling

Food allergies are on the rise and can be deadly. In the U.S. and Canada, labels must note foods that contain the top allergens, gluten, and added sulphites. When something has an added "Gluten-free" label that means that the item does not include any gluten-containing ingredients, although there still may be cross-contamination. An item can be certified gluten-free as long as it has 20 parts-per-million of gluten or less, which is safe for those with celiac disease.

Growing a Healthy Baby as a Vegetarian

I was a vegetarian, and for some years a vegan (strict vegetarian), during my early adult life. I chose this path for a mixture of health, environmental, and ethical reasons. But I do not recommend this for the preconception, pregnancy, and postpartum years. I'm not knocking the power of a plant-based diet. Indeed, I have known and read about people recovering from very serious diseases through radical plant-based diets. Yet, for most of us, the research (and every nutritionist and doctor that I interviewed for this book) suggests that the healthiest diets for growing babies are those that are based primarily on the consumption of lots of fresh, organic vegetables, with a good mix of organic whole grains, fruits, fats, *and* animal products.

If your religious beliefs or ethics require you to be vegetarian, then that is the right choice for you, although I do encourage you to seek guidance in ensuring you and your child are getting enough amino acids, calcium, iron, vitamin B12, omega-3 fatty acids, and good fats in general.

If not, then I urge you to consider including small amounts of animal protein, especially bone broth and fish oil, into your diet. Make sure they are from sources as happy, healthy, and free-ranging as you, yourself, want to be.

It can take extra work to raise your child vegetarian, especially vegan. Here is what you need to know if you are contemplating having a vegetarian baby:

1. First and foremost, a vegan baby should be breastfed for as long as possible (at least a year). There is some concern that the breast milk from vegan moms may lack sufficient DHA, an omega-3 vital for eye and brain development, and taurine (an amino acid). Similarly, postpartum mothers need to be very careful about these levels for their own health and happiness.

2. Babies and young children need cholesterol to build their brains and nerve cells. Egg yolks contain both cholesterol and choline used for healthy brain development. For vegans, cholesterol can be made in the body from healthy saturated fats such as avocado, flax seeds and oil, and coconut oil. But it's not clear that babies can synthesize all the cholesterol they need from vegan sources alone.

3. Children need good-quality fats. Brains are made up of 60 percent fat, more than a third of which is the essential fatty acid DHA. Essential fatty acids are fats that the body can't produce itself. They are found in fish, fish oil, and seaweed, and can be made from olive oil, seeds, and nuts. Read more about fats in the **Essential Nutrients and Where to Find Them** section on pages 43–69.

4. Children need bile to process fat, and taurine plays an essential part in the production and flow of bile. Taurine is also essential in the development and function of the brain and nervous system, kidney development, and the removal of toxins from the body. Taurine can be low in strict vegetarians, as meat, fish, and dairy (and breast milk) are its major sources. Although adults can manufacture some taurine themselves from the essential amino acids methionine and cysteine, newborns cannot. Taurine production can be inhibited by chronic candida, bacterial imbalances, elevated levels of mercury, lead, and cadmium, and exposure to MSG. Urine analysis has shown taurine deficiency in 62 percent of autistic children.

5. Children need protein. The protein in meat, fish, eggs, and milk is usually considered of higher quality, but protein can be gotten from plant

sources such as peas, beans, lentils, chickpeas, seeds, sprouted nuts, and some whole grains. Learn how to cook and prepare and combine foods to maximize their protein content and minimize the anti-nutrients that might inhibit absorption.

6. Common deficiencies to watch for in vegetarian diets are B12, found only in animal foods; vitamins A and D, which are most easily absorbed from meat, fish, eggs, and high-quality butter; minerals such as zinc; and omega-3 fats, which are usually found in fish.

7. Soy can inhibit the absorption of protein and minerals and should be avoided altogether in babies.

The Green Eating Recipe Handbook

• •

The tricks and recipes included in this section will help get even the most reluctant cook started on the joy of home cooking. Many of the recipes are contributed by functional nutritionist Margaret Floyd Barry and her chef husband James Barry of *Eat Naked* and the *Naked Food Cookbook*. Visit them online at www.eatnakednow. com. The rest are adapted from my own kitchen or from favourite cookbooks from the **Further Reading** section on page 226.

Blood-Sugar-Stabilizing Snacks

The trick to balanced blood sugar when snacking is getting lots of good fatty proteins. This might mean eating cheese slices, oysters, sardines, or an avocado, or putting nut butter on apple slices. Or you can try a handful of sprout-soaked nuts or kale chips, a cup of broth, or a fat bomb.

Fat Bombs by Eat Naked

This is a delicious and easy snack that's great for getting those healthy fats important for baby's development and your blood sugar handling. The sauerkraut gives you a little probiotic boost and nice tang. Whitefish caviar is packed with omega-3s and is quite affordable. It's also a little salty, so it balances out the creaminess of the avocado and the tang of the sauerkraut.

This recipe makes one or two snack-size portions, depending on how hungry you are.

Ingredients:
1 avocado
2 tablespoons (18g) raw cultured sauerkraut, either store-bought or homemade
2 teaspoons (11g) whitefish caviar

Directions:
1. Cut avocado in half lengthwise and remove the pit.
2. Add one tablespoon sauerkraut to each half of the avocado in the little hole left from the pit, and place a teaspoon of caviar on top of each.
3. Enjoy! (I just scoop it out with a spoon.)

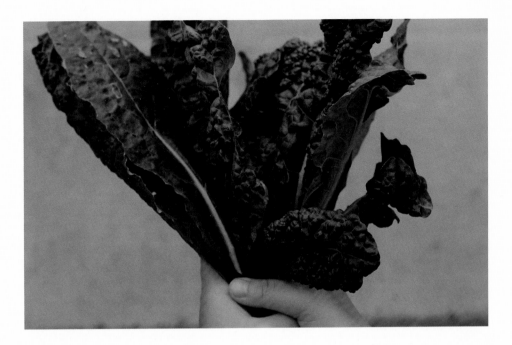

Kale Chips by Eat Naked

Makes 4 servings.

Ingredients:
1 bunch kale, stems cut off and roughly chopped (approximately 3 cups [750ml])
1 tablespoon (15ml) coconut oil, slightly warmed so that it's in liquid form
1⁄4 teaspoon (6g) sea salt, or to taste

Directions:
1. Preheat oven to 400°F (205°C)
2. Place chopped kale in a bowl and drizzle with coconut oil. Using your hands, mix the kale and oil so that the leaves are lightly coated.
3. Spread out the kale on a baking sheet and sprinkle with sea salt to taste.
4. Bake in preheated oven for 5 minutes. Remove tray from oven and stir. Return to oven and continue to cook for 5 to 6 more minutes, or until just slightly browned and crispy.

Soaked Nuts

You can make organic, raw nuts (such as pecans, walnuts, almonds, cashews, or skinless hazelnuts) more digestible and remove the phytotoxins on their skins by placing them in a bowl and covering them with salt water — about 1 cup of nuts to 2 cups of water with just under a tablespoon of salt (I rarely use measuring spoons). Just dissolve the sea salt in the warm water and see that it tastes about as salty as tears or the ocean. After 6 to 12 hours (never soak cashews more than 6 hours), drain the nuts and spread them out on a baking sheet. Place the sheet in a warm spot (130°F to 160°F). A dehydrator, your oven at the lowest temperature, or even on top of a radiator or near a wood-burning stove works well. It will take about 24 hours for them to become completely dry. One time I didn't get my almonds dry enough and they developed mould, a disgusting and expensive mistake.

Probiotic-Rich Foods

Making your own probiotic-rich foods is so simple once you start. You are literally making something from nothing by capturing bacteria from the air to make food that is alive with lots of the good microbes that our guts need and want. Most probiotic-rich food has far more positive bacteria and types than even the best probiotic supplement. All you need to get started is good-quality sea salt or Himalayan salt, filtered water (without chlorine or fluoride, which will inhibit the fermentation), and a few glass jars.

Simple Sauerkraut

Shred cabbage and layer it into a jar along with enough salt to make the final result salty like the sea. A pinch with every layer of cabbage should get you there. Put a rock or something similar on top (not metal) to weigh the sauerkraut down and leave a bit of head room in the jar. The cabbage and salt will produce a brine, and within a few hours there should be enough brine to cover the sauerkraut. If not, add a bit of water and taste to make sure everything is still slightly salty. Leave it for about a week, but check on it every day and push the cabbage under the brine to keep mould from forming. In about a week, you should have slightly bubbly, probiotic-rich sauerkraut. Store in the refrigerator or a cold cellar and enjoy!

Beet Kvass

Ingredients:
2–4 organic beets
1–2 tablespoons (18–36ml) of sea salt
filtered water

Directions:

1. Wash the beets and trim off the leaves and bottoms. Chop into small cubes (don't grate).
2. Place the beets in a large glass jar — the 2-litre size works best.
3. Add the sea salt to taste, to make a slightly salty brine.
4. Fill almost to the top with filtered water, leaving a bit of head room.
5. You can kick-start the kvass by adding a 1/4 cup (60ml) of juice from your prepared sauerkraut (above).
6. Cover the jar tightly and leave it on the counter at room temperature. Check every day to see if it is to your desired taste. This usually takes two to four days.
7. Once it is to your taste, stick in the refrigerator for a couple of days.
8. Drain off the liquid and drink.

You can make it again using the same beets, up to three times. Leave a bit of the liquid in the jar to start your next batch.

Ginger Beer

This is the most complicated of the fermented recipes, but it still isn't that hard — and it's delicious: better tasting and better for you than any soda or most commercially available fermented drinks, such as kombucha. In this recipe, you will start by making what is called a "bug," the probiotic-rich starter, kind of like a sourdough starter.

Make the ginger bug:

Grate a bit of organic ginger with skin into a jar. I use about two inches. Add some water and some unbleached sugar. I sweeten like I salt, by tasting to see if it tastes sweet. Cover the jar with a cloth and leave out. Every day, stir it and add a little more ginger and sugar until the mixture is quite bubbly. This bug can be kept forever. Store it in the refrigerator, where you will occasionally dump a bit of the water out and feed it more sugar and ginger. Just take it out and liven it up before your next use.

Make the ginger beer:

Fill a cooking pot with water (about half of the final volume you want to make). Add finely sliced or grated ginger. Use about 5 to 15 centimetres of ginger root per 2 litres of water in the pot. Bring to a boil and simmer for about 15 minutes. Note: The final mixture should be more gingery than you want it, because it will be diluted. Strain the liquid into a new container and add unrefined sugar to taste, about 2 cups (500ml) per 2 litres of concentrate. Stir and then add cool filtered water until it is the amount and flavour you like. I like to add a bit of lemon juice at this stage as well — again, to taste. The mixture should be brought to room temperature before adding the ginger bug. I usually add 1 cup (250ml) of ginger bug for each 4 litres of liquid, but you can adjust as you like and it will still work. Stir well. Now, you can put the liquid directly into bottles and cover them. Let it sit until it is bubbly, and then bottle it. Be careful: once it is bottled, you can over-carbonate. If you bottle in plastic, you will know when the ginger beer is done because the bottle will get hard and bulge slightly. If you, like me, prefer to bottle in glass, you must be much more careful. One way is to do at least one bottle in plastic to gauge how the others are doing. I have had serious and scary explosions occur, where glass flew everywhere from over-carbonation. Once you put the bottles in the refrigerator, the fermenting process will slow down, but still enjoy it within a few weeks.

Simple, Nourishing Meals

One of Margaret Floyd Barry's tips is to remember to front load your day and each meal with all-important fats and proteins. This will aid in digestion and stabilizing blood sugar. You might start your day with two fried eggs served with greens or simple breakfast porridge served with a generous dollop of organic, grass-fed butter. Add a cup of bone broth as an appetizer to lunch or dinner, or make the meal a nutrient-packed soup with salad. Here are a few recipes to get you started.

Simple Breakfast Porridge

The typical breakfast cereal is made from grains that have been extruded, which destroys the fatty acids, vitamins, and amino acids in them, making them hard to digest and even toxic. These grains aren't soaked, obviously, so the phytic acid hasn't been reduced. This isn't to mention the problems associated with non-organic cereals, which are often genetically modified to have even more pesticides than usual. Hot breakfast cereals can be a more nutritious alternative.

The simplest way to prepare this is to take your favourite grain, such as organic rolled oats, and soak them overnight to make them more digestible. Soak 1 cup (156g) of oats in a cup of warm water with 2 tablespoons (30g) of plain yogourt (or whey, if you have it, or lemon juice if you are allergic to dairy). In the morning add another cup of water and cook. It takes about 10 minutes on medium-low heat. Add in a lot of butter at the end and you are ready to go. Top as you like. My kids prefer this served with pure, organic maple syrup, but I eat mine with salt, pepper, and some nuts and seeds. There are two of us in my family who can't digest oats, so we have done this same recipe with quinoa and spelt flakes.

For a more protein-packed breakfast porridge, you can make your own blend and tailor it to make it gluten-free or whatever you prefer. Use approximately 1 cup of each grain. I recommend any, or all, of the following: yellow split peas or red lentils, barley, spelt, rice, quinoa, millet, and oats. Combine your grains and blend or food process until medium smooth and well mixed. Store in a container in your refrigerator until you are ready to use for making breakfast porridge. Use the basic recipe above to cook: 1 cup of the grain mixture soaked overnight in 1 cup (250ml) of warm water with 2 tablespoons (30g) of yogourt (or other). Add an additional cup of water before cooking the next morning. Depending on the blend, it may take longer than oatmeal (lentils and brown rice are slow). Cook for 15 to 35 minutes on medium-low heat until to desired doneness.

Fish Broth

This is a great recipe adapted by Floyd Barry from Sally Fallon Morell's excellent cookbook *Nourishing Traditions*.

Ingredients:
2 tablespoons (28g) organic butter
2 onions, roughly chopped
1 carrot, roughly chopped
1/2 cup (125ml) dry white wine
3 or 4 whole fish carcasses, including heads, of non-oily fish such as sole, turbot, rockfish, or snapper
about 3 litres of cold filtered water
1/4 cup (60ml) vinegar
a few sprigs of fresh thyme
a few sprigs of fresh parsley
1 bay leaf

Directions:
1. Melt butter in a large stainless steel pot.
2. Add the vegetables and cook very gently, for about 30 minutes, until soft.
3. Add wine and bring to a boil.
4. Add fish carcasses and cover with cold, filtered water. Add vinegar.
5. Bring to a boil, covered, and skim off the scum and impurities as they rise to the top.
6. Tie herbs together and add to the pot. Reduce heat to absolute lowest, and simmer for at least 4 hours or as long as 24 hours.
7. Remove carcasses with tongs or a slotted spoon and strain the liquid into pint-size storage containers for refrigeration or freezing. Chill well in the

refrigerator and remove any congealed fat before transferring to the freezer for long-term storage.

Simple Fish Soup

Fish stock can be used as the broth for just about any recipe, from a substitution for water when making rice or barley to the base of clam chowder or vegetable soup. My favourite recipe is for making a simple Asian noodle soup. I cook the noodles separately, heat the broth, add my favourite vegetables (usually carrots, bok choy, green onions, and a few slices of cucumber) and then serve with freshly chopped cilantro or basil. I adjust the flavour as needed by using organic bouillon, flavoured vinegars, or herbs.

Chicken Bone Broth

Use a whole chicken (with the feet if you can get them). Remove the internal organs and cut off the meat for other recipes or for adding to the final soup. (I've also used the carcass after baking a whole chicken.) Place the chicken or chicken pieces into a large stainless steel pot with 4 litres (or a bit more) of cold water and 2 tablespoons (30ml) of apple cider vinegar. Let stand 1 hour. Add vegetables. I keep a bag of vegetable scraps in my freezer, so I just add that. For a more consistent taste, add one large onion, two carrots, three celery stalks, and four cloves of garlic, all coarsely chopped. Bring to a boil and remove any scum with a slotted spoon as it comes to the top. Reduce heat and simmer for 3 to 24 hours. Chefs tend to vote for less time, but some nutritionists say the longer the better. Right before turning off the heat, add a bunch of parsley. Allow to sit and cool. Strain the stock into a large pot or bowl. Put into the refrigerator and allow to cool completely. A layer of fat will congeal on the top. Remove this before using or separating the broth into containers to freeze. I often turn about a quarter of it into chicken broth cubes by pouring it into ice cube trays, freezing, and then storing in freezer bags so I can just grab one or two as needed.

Chicken Soup

Chop and cook one onion in a soup pot. Add slices of chicken (raw or cooked). Pour in about 1 litre of homemade broth. Add your choice of vegetables, such as two carrots and three stalks of celery, both finely sliced. Cook on medium heat until vegetables are tender, about 30 minutes to 1 hour. Add salt and pepper to taste.

Boosted Burgers by Eat Naked

Organ meat is nutrient-dense and really healthy for pregnant and nursing mamas. The Barrys have a local farmer who sells a product he calls "boost" — ground, grass-fed bison with 10 percent beef liver ground into it. This is a tasty way to sneak liver into your diet without anyone noticing. Not everyone is as lucky as the Barrys to have such a forward-thinking farmer nearby, so they developed this recipe for the rest of us! Makes 4 servings.

Ingredients:
2 oz (60g) frozen beef liver, still frozen
1 lb (1/2 kg) ground grass-fed beef or bison
1 teaspoon (5ml) dried oregano
1 teaspoon (5ml) paprika
1 tablespoon (14g) coconut oil or lard from pastured pork

Directions:
1. Grate or mince frozen liver into a large mixing bowl. **Pro tip:** Since most beef liver is sold in sizes significantly larger than these small portions, try cutting the liver into 60 gram portions when you first buy it *before* freezing.
2. Add the ground meat and spices. Stir to mix well.
3. Divide the ground meat mixture into 8 equal portions and roll each into a ball. Set aside.
4. Heat the coconut oil or lard in a large, heavy-bottomed fry pan (such as a cast iron skillet) over medium-high heat. When the skillet is hot, place the meat balls in it, using a spatula to press down on them to make patty-shaped.
5. Cook for 3–4 minutes on one side until nicely browned, then flip to cook on the other side. Cook for another 3–4 minutes or until just cooked through if you like it pink in the middle, or a little longer if you like them more well done.
6. Serve with your favourite hamburger fixings, such as lettuce, fresh farmers' market tomatoes, homemade pickles, or mushrooms sautéed in lots of butter.

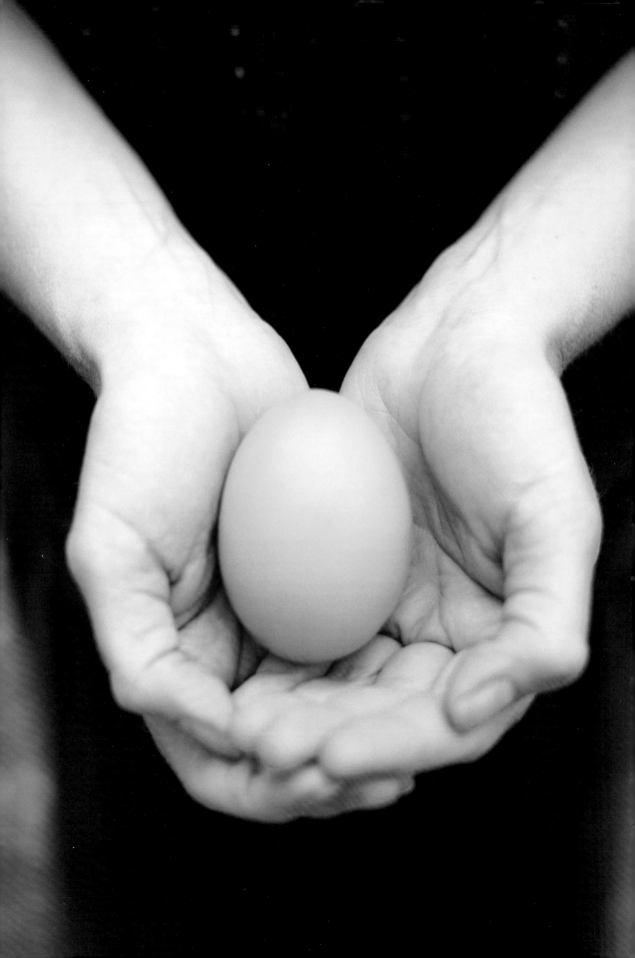

Greening the Growing Fetus

• •

It was only a generation ago that we thought the growing fetus was entirely protected by the placenta. At that time, we had little idea that toxins, including drugs and alcohol, could reach the growing child. We have since learned that many do.

I once read in a dusty old book that pregnancy was one of the only cures for lead poisoning. In it, they described how a pregnant mother could watch her teeth regain their normal colour as the baby-to-be absorbed the lead.

We learned the hard way that the placenta wasn't much of a barrier at all. One of the bitterest lessons came in the form of the sedative thalidomide, marketed to help with the effects of morning sickness during pregnancy in the late 1950s and 1960s. Soon after it appeared, doctors began to notice a startling rise in severe birth defects in women who had used the drug during pregnancy. It remained available in Canada months after it was removed from use in West Germany and the U.K.

The U.S. was protected from the worst of this disaster by a Canadian woman, scientist, and medical doctor, Dr. Frances Oldham Kelsey. She had just begun working for the FDA at the time and refused to give the drug her blessing for use in the United States despite "relentless pressures" from the drug's manufacturer. She insisted that, despite its popularity in England, there was not enough evidence to prove it was safe for use during pregnancy. This British Columbia–born doctor was tenacious in the face of pressure, in part because she had participated in research earlier in her career that demonstrated some drugs could cross the placenta and affect unborn children.

The Research

The placenta is a mother's protective impulse turned physical. The placenta starts developing at the same time as the embryo. In the fifth week of gestation, the umbilical cord develops and attaches the embryo's abdomen to the placenta. Inside

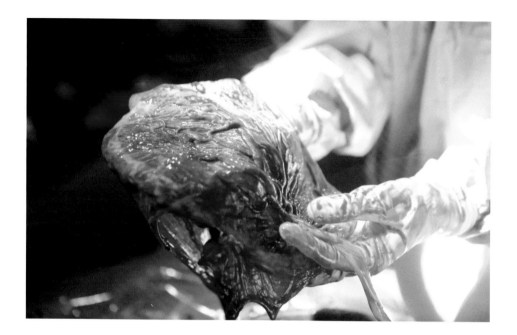

the placenta, the baby is surrounded by amniotic fluid held within the amniotic sac. The outer layer of the amniotic sac is part of the placenta, and the placenta attaches to the uterus. The amniotic fluid is made by the mother's blood plasma and is absorbed by the fetus's skin.

The placenta serves two primary functions. One is to deliver nutrients from the mother's blood to the fetus and produce hormones, including estrogen and progesterone. These hormones are used for the fetus's development and to help prepare the mother for delivery and lactation. The other function is protective. It protects the blood of the child from the blood of the mother. This is how a child can have a different blood type from the mother. It is also how the baby is protected from certain diseases and even some toxins. The placenta also allows waste from the baby's developing metabolism, such as carbon dioxide, to move back through the umbilical cord to the mother's bloodstream for clean-up.

Enter into this picture of biological bliss the toxins found in the environment today and things get more complicated. Yet our basic biology still wants to protect us and our growing babies. We can help this biological impulse by reducing our exposure to toxins, minimizing drug use during pregnancy, and providing good, healthy nourishment, which helps keep our natural systems working as effectively as possible.

"Forbidden" Foods That Needn't Be Forsaken

It isn't that surprising to me to discover that the placenta is actually well adapted to protect the developing baby from diseases, including most viruses and food-borne illnesses. Thus, contracting E. coli from a fast-food hamburger while pregnant is likely to be very uncomfortable, but it isn't likely to cause harm to the baby. There are exceptions, however, and these exceptions are at the root of why North Americans are relatively uptight about certain foods in pregnancy compared to their European peers. The exceptions include *Listeria monocytogenes* (often associated with soft, raw cheeses and lunch meats) and *Salmonella enterica* (associated with undercooked meat and eggs), both of which can cause harm in the unborn fetus.

The risk, however, is extremely low. A scientific paper published in the *Canadian Family Physician* explained that women need not avoid most of the foods we've come to fear, such as those soft cheeses, as long as they are from a safe and reputable source. Foods that can be enjoyed with caution include

- **Runny eggs.** The take-away on undercooked foods, such as runny eggs, and contracting salmonella is that the risk is minuscule — an average of 1 in 20,000 — and that pregnant women are at no greater risk than the rest of the non-pregnant population. The risk of contracting salmonella from undercooked eggs is considered even smaller from organic, pastured eggs. Cooking the egg thoroughly removes the risk.
- **Raw fish and other seafood.** The study authors say go ahead and eat sushi or undercooked seafood as long as it is from a reputable establishment, has been stored properly, and is consumed fresh. Any infections that might happen from seafood tend to be limited to the GI tract, so while they may be uncomfortable, they won't harm the fetus. **The authors do caution against the consumption of high-mercury fish and shellfish, including tuna.**
- **Raw honey.** The authors also state that there is no known risk to the fetus from honey that might contain botulinum toxin and that the average healthy women need not avoid raw honey during pregnancy.

All in all, most foods are safe for women to consume during pregnancy as long as they are from safe, reputable sources. When I was pregnant, I chose to eat the way I always have: fried eggs with runny yellows; raw, non-homogenized milk; wild-caught salmon; and unpasteurized honey. I do my utmost to be sure about my sources, finding products that are organic, locally sourced, pasture-raised, or wild-caught. You can learn what to look for in healthy sources in the **Organic-ize Your Diet** section in the previous chapter.

Why the Placenta Doesn't Better Protect Baby from Toxins

Just as it intuitively makes sense that the placenta would have evolved to protect a fetus from most illnesses, I'm also not surprised that the placenta is unable to better protect a baby from many of the 42 billion pounds of industrial chemicals imported or manufactured every day in North America. Perhaps one day the placenta will evolve to parse the heavy metals from the calcium before passing them on to the baby-to-be, but as of now most toxins cross into the developing fetus. Some, like mercury, concentrate in the baby-to-be. The end result is that a baby born today in Canada will be born pre-polluted with more than 130 different known or suspected toxins.

Your baby is not alone in her exposure levels: we all share the air and the water. Indeed, some of the most pristine areas of the world — like remote regions of Arctic Canada — have the highest concentrations of industrial toxins. These are areas thousands of kilometres from the nearest factory or coal-powered plant, but have nevertheless become receptacles of known poisons thanks to trade winds and ocean currents. There are things that parents can do to protect our children and that we can all do to protect our future generations from the worst of these toxins. It helps to know *when* a child is the most vulnerable and *what* toxins are of greatest concern.

The *When*: Critical Windows of Exposure

When I was pregnant, I had a day-by-day pregnancy journal that apprised me of what was happening in my womb. One day, near the end of the first month, the book announced, "By the end of this month, your baby will have completed a period of growth that involves the greatest size and physical changes of its lifetime. In five days, it will be 10,000 times larger than the fertilized egg, although in actuality not much bigger than a grain of rice." And on day 140, it said, "If your baby is a female, her uterus is completely formed and has just undergone its most rapid period of growth."

All healthy babies-to-be develop along similar lines and similar time frames (give or take a few days or weeks). The developing baby might have a bit more of a particular nutritional need or be especially affected by exposures to toxins or drugs, depending on what is happening at that moment with his development. One example of this is with thalidomide, the drug mentioned earlier that was prescribed as a treatment for morning sickness. When it was given to women in the fourth and ninth weeks of pregnancy, the drug caused severe birth defects, while women who took it outside that time experienced little risk of those same effects.

Baby teeth might also hold a key to understanding more about windows of exposure and the effects of different environmental toxins. Teeth form rings as they grow — kind of like trees — that reveal daily information about the totality of health-affecting exposures known as the "exposome." By studying teeth, we can better understand the relationship between particular exposures at particular times and the resultant health outcomes. There are studies underway now using teeth biomarkers to understand more about causes of childhood leukemia — which is not genetic and, thus, is considered environmental — as well as adult chronic illnesses such as Alzheimer's and heart disease. This research can help scientists, doctors, and parents-to-be figure out the human effects of the increased number of chemicals we are exposed to and how to prioritize protective actions during pregnancy.

The *What*: Chemicals to Be Avoided Prenatally

Industrial chemicals have made their way into nearly every aspect of modern life, from our shampoo to our sheets. Understanding what things are called, where they are lurking, and why they are bad helps us in avoiding them. It also helps parents understand why it's worth it to buy an organic apple or avoid a ripped sofa.

- **Heavy metals** such as arsenic, lead, cadmium, and mercury are a problem because they can be stored in our bodies and easily pass through the placenta, where they can particularly affect the developing brain. They are found in beauty care products and in the fatty tissue of certain animals, in particular fish. Luckily there are safer options, such as greener beauty care and eating smaller, wild-caught fish.
- **Persistent organic pollutants (POPs)** are dangerous because they can be very toxic and long-lasting. In particular they can affect the hormones and the developing brain, and many have been linked with cancers. POPs include certain pesticides (such as DDT and hexachlorabenzene), flame retardants (including PBDEs and Tris), water- and stain-resistors (such as PFOA and PFOS), and by-products from industrial processes (such as dioxin and PCBs). These can end up in the food chain by being added directly as a pesticide or indirectly through contamination of the water and flesh of other animals. You can reduce your exposure to POPs by making those healthy food choices discussed in the last chapter, and also by greening your home and beauty care routine.
- **Volatile organic compounds (VOCs)** readily release into the environment and can cause a range of health concerns from headaches to organ damage after they are inhaled and make their way into your bloodstream. They are commonly found in paints, solvents, highway traffic, cigarette smoke, building materials, household cleaning products, and beauty care items. There are many ways to avoid the worst of the VOCs — for instance by avoiding cigarette smoke and greening your home. Keep reading to learn more.
- **Pesticides** aren't always so persistent, but can still be harmful because of their pervasiveness. Their residues can be found in most conventionally grown foods and most of our drinking water, and they can be added to products such as antibacterial hand soaps and cleaning products. Learning to read labels can help you avoid these unwanted ingredients.
- **Plastics** in almost all cases have the ability to interfere with developing hormones. The worst of the plasticizers, including phthalates, BPA, melamine, PVC, and polystyrene, can largely be avoided by keeping them away from your kitchen and not using them in food preparation or storage.

Learn more about these chemicals and where they are found in the **Green Mama-to-Be*ware*** appendix.

More *What*: Drugs and Exposures to Approach with Caution During Pregnancy

When my grandmother was pregnant, it was possible that a doctor would enter the room smoking a cigarette, and women were even allowed to smoke in some maternity wards. Indeed, a stiff drink to wash down the diet pills prescribed by the doctor wasn't uncommon then either.

We've come a long way from those times, but many of the substances we encounter in our daily living can still harm a baby-to-be. Some of these, like tobacco, are better understood, but others, like acetaminophen, we are just beginning to understand. We do know enough to be cautious about the following commonly used drugs.

The chemicals in **cigarettes** are among the most studied prenatal toxins, and e-cigarettes may be just as bad. As recently as 2007, it was reported that up to 15 percent of pregnant women smoke, and many millions more are exposed to secondhand smoke, which may be just as dangerous. Its detrimental effects to a growing baby-to-be and even future grand-babies-to-be include miscarriage, reduced birth weight, and an increased risk for chronic diseases, respiratory disease, asthma, allergies, cancer, cognitive impairment, and behavioural disorders, including aggression, ADHD, major depression disorder, substance abuse, and other externalizing disorders. Cigarette smoke contains more than 4,000 chemicals, of which more than 40 are known carcinogens and at least some of which — such as nicotine — do cross the placenta, where they can show up in higher concentrations in the baby than in the mother.

A number of my friends and family members have finally kicked their smoking habits with the help of e-cigarettes. While less is known about the effects of e-cigarettes on health because there has not been time to do adequate research, early studies suggest that they may not be much healthier than regular old cigarettes. The FDA published a review in 2014 cautioning against the many known and potential toxins that they contain and can release in their vapours, including nitrosamines, aldehydes, metals, VOCs, nanoparticles, and nicotine. Indeed, the class one — known human carcinogen — formaldehyde can be up to 15 times higher in e-cig vapour than in cigarette smoke. Researchers and health organizations caution that even the second-hand vapours should not be considered safe for fetuses, babies, or children.

As with many toxins, some researchers say there is no safe level of **alcohol** when it comes to protecting the fetus. Your doctor will likely say this as well, for two reasons. One, it is known that fetal alcohol spectrum disorder (FASD) can cause irreparable harm to a baby, including physical deformities, mental handicaps, learning disabilities, and behavioural disorders. Two, because there is simply no ethical way to do controlled experiments involving alcohol and pregnant women.

We don't know much about what a moderate alcohol level does to the fetus. It is during the first trimester that alcohol consumption is most likely to lead to physical deformities. We also know from sibling comparison studies that even light to moderate drinking can lead to some behavioural problems.

Can You Tox-Out Toxins?

Can we detoxify ourselves? That's the question behind *ToxIn ToxOut*, the sequel to Bruce Lourie and Rick Smith's bestselling book *Slow Death by Rubber Duck*. In it, the intrepid authors exposed themselves to numerous everyday items: BPA and pesticides in foods, phthalates and fire retardants found in furniture, and triclosan and phthalates in skincare products. All the while, they tested their blood and urine and found, yup, the levels of toxins in their bodies increased noticeably. Then they tried to figure out if it was possible to get these toxins out of their bodies, and how.

In short, "A lot of detox therapies just aren't that effective," warns Smith. Chelation was one of the "big hitter" techniques they tested and found could work to reduce some of those longer-lasting toxins such as aluminum, mercury, and lead. Chelation involves using an intravenous agent that travels through the bloodstream, grabbing onto minerals and metals and binding with them. These bound minerals and metals then move through the digestive system and out of the body through the urine. Doctors have used chelation to help treat diseases including arthritis, autism, fibromyalgia, and Parkinson's, and even as an alternative to heart bypass surgery. It can be risky, though, because chelation binds with minerals as well as heavy metals. Chelation might be something to consider if you are having trouble conceiving or when preparing for a pregnancy (in consultation with a medical professional) about a year before trying to get pregnant. Chelation is *not* on the menu for someone who is already pregnant, within the few months leading up to conception, or breastfeeding.

Everyday detoxification methods for children and mamas-to-be that were proven to work include sweating, pooping, peeing, and all of the things tied to creating "beautiful pathways of elimination," as nutritionist Margaret Floyd Barry puts it. They also tested and confirmed that you could successfully limit and lower toxin levels in children by doing all those great Green Mama things, like feeding them fresh organic food, improving indoor air quality, getting children outside more, and encouraging them to exercise. The best thing, of course, "is [to] try to shield them from these chemicals in the first place," says Smith.

There is another complexity in all of this: FASD seems to be affected by genetics. That's right; alcohol consumption of the mother affects some babies more than others. The genetics of both mother *and child* seem to play a part in this.

Over-the-counter products for pain relief can also be toxic to the fetus. For many years, the go-to medicine for pregnant women was acetaminophen, better known as Tylenol. That changed in 2014, when the Danish National Cohort Study looked at 64,322 live births and found that mothers who used acetaminophen during pregnancy were more likely to have children with ADHD, ADHD-like behaviours, and hyperkinetic disorders. The more frequent the use, the higher the chance of the outcome. No trimesters were safe, and exposure in more trimesters also increased risk.

Other over-the-counter pain relievers seem to be no safer. Doctors and midwives have warned against the use of painkillers such as ibuprofen, diclofenac, and other non-steroid anti-inflammatory drugs (NSAIDs) because they more than double the risk of miscarriage in the first 20 weeks and are associated with low birth weights when used in the second trimester and asthma when used in the second or third trimester. You can find other more natural remedies to help with occasional pain in the **Natural Pregnancy Handbook** following this chapter.

Caffeine is one of the most popular mood-altering drugs. It can help a person feel more awake and energetic by stimulating a number of hormones in the brain, including dopamine, and it blocks adenosine, a brain chemical associated with feelings of drowsiness. The more caffeine a person drinks, the more a person requires. Unfortunately, caffeine is not so good for your baby. It's been shown to cross the placenta to the baby-to-be, where the baby's developing metabolism is ill-equipped to handle the effects, which include keeping him awake. Caffeine has been linked to reduced fertility in men and women, an increased chance of miscarriage, and low birth weights, and it may even be linked to preterm birth and some birth defects. In short, scientists say there is no proven safe limit of caffeine use during pregnancy.

Most healthcare practitioners advise that you reduce your levels to below 200 mg a day while pregnant. That equals one cup of organic coffee, up to a few cups of black or green tea, or a couple of pieces of dark chocolate. I'd suggest going decaf (but read about the importance of going organic when you do that, or try decaffeinating your own organic tea at home). Don't drink your tea or coffee on an empty stomach either; it's far better for your blood sugar (and your baby) to drink it after one of those healthy, blood-sugar-smart meals discussed in the previous chapter.

Avoid unnecessary **ultrasounds.** Ninety-nine percent of women in Canada will have an ultrasound during their pregnancy. While the procedure is considered safe for mother and baby, there are some risks. A growing number of studies are showing that ultrasound may cause harm in the growing fetus because of the relatively high amount of heat and sound that they produce. While heat and sound don't seem particularly disturbing, the research suggests we may have underestimated their effects on the fetus, for which high heat can lead to central nervous system damage. (This is why we aren't supposed to submerge for long periods of time in super-hot tubs or saunas, particularly in early pregnancy when the organs and central nervous system are forming.) The sound inside the woman's uterus during an ultrasound was compared to a "subway train coming into a station," according to a 2011 study in which the researchers put a microphone that detects sound waves underwater into a woman's uterus during an ultrasound.

Dr. Bethany Hays, an obstetrician with more than 30 years of experience, says she sees ultrasounds being over-prescribed. Guidelines indicate that they should be limited to one or two per pregnancy when medically indicated. But what is meant by *medically indicated*? Hays says situations when a woman might want an ultrasound include early in the pregnancy if there is pain or bleeding (to ensure the pregnancy is forming in the uterus); if the mother doesn't have clear menstrual dates before 12 weeks to nail down a delivery date; as an alternative to other genetic screening at 18 to 20 weeks (she cautions it cannot be used effectively for genetic screening if done any earlier); in cases where fundal height or fetal growth are in question; or if you are concerned about amniotic fluid in a high-risk pregnancy. The Society of Obstetricians and Gynecologists of Canada have guidelines around the use of ultrasound in pregnancy. They caution that ultrasounds should not be used to just determine the sex of the baby and that "if your health-care provider recommends that you have an ultrasound, make sure you know why it is needed, the risks that may be involved, and how it will be done."

Little Things Matter

Dr. Bruce Lanphear — toxin scientist, medical doctor, and dad — reminds us that "not all chemicals are bad." Yet it only takes a tiny dose of the bad chemicals to "have a lifelong impact on children." The amounts seen in children today, though so minuscule they are measured in parts per billion (ppb), are causing serious effects, including loss of IQ points. The combined total can be substantial in one child and even more substantial in the population as a whole. "Children with more exposure to toxins won't reach the same cognitive abilities as those exposed to less," says Lanphear. "Little shifts in children's IQ scores [have] a big impact on the number of children challenged."

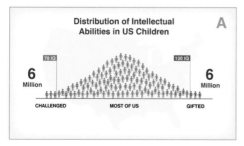

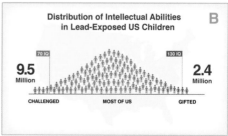

The Beautiful, Vulnerable Brain

"[The brain] makes us who we are," says Dr. Bruce Lanphear. It's so important that it has its own built-in biological protection system: the blood-brain barrier. Like the placenta, however, the blood-brain barrier is really more like a porous protection system. Large molecules, molecules that have a high electrical charge, and molecules with low lipid (fat) content do not pass readily through the blood-brain barrier. This means that it can help create a more consistent environment for the brain, protecting it from many foreign substances and hormones and neurotransmitters that travel through the rest of the body. The blood-brain barrier is not fully developed at birth and does not function as well when coupled with high blood pressure, infection, or inflammation or when exposed to high concentrations of chemicals in the blood, microwaves, or radiation.

The brain is particularly vulnerable to the effects of toxin exposure. It is susceptible for two reasons. The brain develops over such an extended period of time (in other words, it has many windows of exposure) beginning soon after conception and continuing for at least two years after birth. The brain is also susceptible because of the rapid rate at which it develops. Rapid growth creates added vulnerability. "This is why chemotherapy works on cancer," Lanphear explains. The chemotherapy drugs kill the rapidly growing cancer cells, but they don't affect the slow-developing cells of healthy tissue. Toxins can target the nervous system and brain because they are particularly drawn to the rapidly developing brain tissue.

If contributing factors of conditions such as ADHD and autism spectrum disorders can be removed, says Lanphear, "then which and why some children are more susceptible ceases to matter." The key to prevention, then, is to identify any environmental risk factor and remove it. And there have been successes. Lead has been removed from gasoline and paints and children's products. In turn, levels of lead (and also banned substances such as DDT, PBDEs, and PCBs) are diminishing in our children as those chemicals are phased out of use.

And while our science and government regulations may be lacking in North America, there is a silver lining. Citizens, many of them parents, are increasingly demanding safer products and getting companies to change. This citizen pressure has led to victories from Johnson & Johnson's promise to phase out formaldehyde-releasing ingredients from its baby products to Whole Foods leading the charge on removing the worst cosmetics and food additives from its shelves. Similar to what happened with the consumer outrage over BPA, these are victories for citizen action.

Canadians can make a difference by asking better questions of the research that is presented on all chemicals and consumer products, avoiding products with unproven ingredients, asking companies to change their formulations, and asking their elected officials and governing bodies to take greater action on protecting human health from everyday toxins.

It all starts here. A new baby is a new opportunity to mother not just this new life, but also life in general. That instinct you have that things aren't quite what they say they are is probably right. Your parenting instincts will only grow stronger, fuelled by a better understanding of the science, your own observations, and a power to ask more of those who represent you and market to you.

How to Get Everyday Toxins Out of Your Pregnancy

Babies, especially while still in utero, are unable to adequately eliminate the toxins to which they are exposed. However, it is possible to reduce their exposure to potentially harmful chemicals by taking greater care in what you eat, drink, breath in, and rub on; avoiding or lessening your exposure to everyday chemicals that have the potential to cross the placenta and provide additional stress on the growing baby; and enhancing your own natural pathways of elimination. Here are a series of action steps listed from ♥♥♥ (biggest impact, and possibly more work) to ♥ (quick and easy) to help you get those nasty toxins out of your pregnancy.

1. ♥♥♥ **Eliminate the big-hitter chemicals and drugs.** If you are reading this book, then you certainly care about growing the healthiest child possible. If you are still smoking cigarettes (or even using e-cigarettes) or drinking in excess, then it is clearly because it is out of your control. For the health of your child and your grandchildren, this is the most important battle you can take on. No amount of organic food and skincare will undo the negative effects of these routine exposures. That doesn't mean these other things don't matter; it's just that as you now know from everything else you have read, two goods can't undo one bad when it comes to toxin exposure and a growing fetus.

   Nearly everybody in my family of origin has been a smoker and tried everything to quit. When nothing else worked, they found help through acupuncture, hypnotism, and diet. Try everything; the stakes are high. Similarly, alcohol addiction is not something most people want to discuss, especially when pregnant. Guilt is not a good motivator, according to my research and experience. Hope, however, is a great motivator. You should know, then, that it isn't too late for your child to benefit from you tackling your addictions. As I have mentioned, my family of origin has suffered greatly through all kinds of drug addictions, and I have seen the healing power ripple down through the generations when a person — even if that person is a grandparent — faces their addictions, whether to alcohol, tobacco, caffeine, work, or even cellphones.

2. ♥♥♥ **Organic-ize your diet and your kitchen.** A nutrient-rich diet is the most important tool in supporting your body's natural ability to eliminate toxins. Eating organic (see the previous chapter for more on this) has also been shown to significantly reduce your exposure to pesticide residue. Continue the good work by keeping **plasticizers (including BPA, phthalates, and more) and water-resistant and non-stick coatings** out of your storage containers, food packaging, pots, and cooking utensils.

   While it is not possible for most of us to completely eliminate plastics from our lives, we can certainly reduce our exposure where it matters the most. All plastics have the potential to release hormone-mimicking chemicals into our food. This includes those items labelled BPA-free, which can still leach other compounds.

   Eating and drinking food from cans is thought to be the largest contributor to our body burden of BPA. I would especially avoid fatty or acidic foods packed in cans, because they can leach more of the chemical into themselves. Instead of buying foods in cans, fresh and frozen foods are a far better option, both from a nutrient perspective as well as from a toxin perspective (and most often a cost perspective).

   When storing food or buying take-out, use glass or stainless steel. Avoid plastics, including plastic wrap, especially for hot foods or foods that will be heated. When this isn't possible, such as when getting take-out, I'd choose just about anything over Styrofoam, especially if the item is hot or acidic.

   Get rid of non-stick and water-resistant cups, wrap, and cookware. You can save money and potential chemical exposure by going with cast iron, ceramic, stainless steel, titanium, or glass pots and pans. For all those water-resistant slick packages, follow the plastic guidelines: the hotter, more fatty, or more acidic, the more nasty chemicals can leach out of the packaging and into the food. I'd ditch the microwave popcorn or the cook-in-bag rice at all costs, but might still buy parsnip chips in a bag with a similar glossy mix of chemicals.

3. ♥♥♥ **Get toxins out of your skincare regime and indoor air.** Learn more about doing this in the next two chapters!

4. ♥♥ **If you are getting the flu shot while pregnant, ensure it is the preservative-free version.** Preservative-free (mercury-free) inactivated flu shots are available for pregnant women. These are packaged and sold as a single-use injection (hence no need for a preservative). Press the point! No amount of mercury exposure is proven safe for pregnant mothers and babies.

5. ♥♥ **When getting dental work, avoid amalgam fillings.** Pregnant women and children in Canada are still routinely exposed to mercury in amalgam dental fillings — despite warnings about its being "extremely toxic" issued by the American Society of Dental Surgeons as early as 1845. Mercury is released from amalgam fillings as vapour, through chewing, brushing, and steady wear and tear. Much of the developed world, including much of the European Union, has entirely or partially restricted the use of amalgam fillings, particularly in pregnant women and in children. Health Canada has issued warnings that it may not be advisable to use amalgam fillings in children and pregnant women, but they continue to be the most common type of filling used in Canada today and are also routinely used in the United States.

6. ♥♥ **Get your pathways of natural elimination working.** The previous chapter had a lot of tips on getting your digestion moving. You can get yourself sweating through gentle exercise and warm baths, pee out more toxins by drinking more water, and ensure you're getting good nutrition.

    Nutritionist Margaret Floyd Barry recommends oil pulling, and while there is no proof that it removes toxins, there is evidence to show it reduces gingivitis. So pull away! Oil pulling is the process of taking edible oil and swishing it around your mouth and teeth for about 20 minutes or so and then spitting it out along with anything it "pulls" from your body. I used to do this in the car on the way to work, and besides being a safe way to gently detox while pregnant, it can also make your teeth brighter and your breath fresher.

7. ♥♥ **Decrease your caffeine intake.** Caffeine is a drug, and there is no proven safe level for a fetus. If you are in the habit of drinking sodas or energy drinks, try replacing them with the probiotic-rich homemade ginger beer (see page 67), or substitute with drinks that contain less caffeine and sugar and more probiotics, such as kefir, water kefir, or kombucha. If you have a habit of drinking coffee, try replacing it with certified organic decaffeinated coffee. The organic certification will protect you from the worst of the chemicals found in the coffee and from the chemically intensive

decaffeination process as well. Or replace it with a cup of black or green tea that you decaffeinate at home (learn how in the previous chapter) or with a cup of herbal pregnancy tea (recipes to follow).

8. ♥♥ **Filter your water.** I recommend a more involved system than a Brita pitcher filter, but even it is far less expensive and far better for you and the environment than bottled water. A really good water filtration system will cost more upfront but will last longer and filter more toxins, and most can be tailored to filter fluoride. There is a growing body of research to suggest that fluoride, a chemical added to the public water supply in much of the U.S. and Canada, may interfere with healthy body functioning and interfere with brain function. Fluoride accumulates in the body, particularly in the bones and pineal gland and the amount in bones increases over a lifetime, with children taking more into their bones than adults. Fluoride also crosses the placenta. Its linked with slowing down the time it takes for teeth to appear, which increases risk of decay. It is also associated with the tooth discolouration called dental fluorosis, now estimated to affect 41 percent of American children.

9. ♥ **Save the ultrasound for when it is medically necessary.** I know; I loved the security I felt from seeing the baby growing inside me and having the doctor say, "Everything looks great!" Just remember that those ultrasounds come with a risk, and it's equally satisfying to minimize that risk. Always ask your healthcare provider why an ultrasound is needed, and then do your own research to see how legitimate that need is and if you can wait. If you were to get just one ultrasound, I'd recommend doing it during that 18- to 20-week window, when the ultrasound can be used in lieu of a number of other tests often prescribed in early pregnancy, many with high rates of error.

10. ♥ **Stop dry cleaning.** The dry-cleaning process exposes workers, those who live nearby, and you when you wear the clothes to one of the nastiest, most persistent toxins there is: perchlorates (PERC). PERCs can affect the endocrine system and is linked with breast cancer. If you wear dry-clean-only clothes for work (or because you are Princess Kate), then you will be happy to know there is a safe alternative to dry cleaning called wet cleaning, and there is almost certainly a wet cleaner in your town.

11. ♥ **Avoid over-the-counter medicines such as painkillers in pregnancy.** As the new research on acetaminophen shows, substances long assumed to be safe are often under-researched. I advise trying the natural, food-based,

or time-tested remedies first. If something is largely food-based (such as herbal tea), then our bodies are usually able to handle it through normal systems of detoxification. Synthesized chemicals — whether in the form of drugs or chemicals or super-concentrated herbal oils — can "outsmart" the body's ability to properly and safely handle them, so it is more likely to make it across the placenta to your baby. That's great if you are trying to treat the baby chemically, but not so great if you are trying to treat the mother without experimenting on the baby-to-be as well. Use natural remedies instead of pharmaceuticals for treating normal pregnancy-related issues such as nausea, swelling, and varicose veins. **Read on for suggestions for gentle herbal teas, homeopathic remedies, and aromatherapy solutions.**

12. ♥ **Develop a gentle exercise routine,** such as yoga, water aerobics (preferably not in a chlorinated pool), Pilates, or walking or hiking, all of which help to keep your natural pathways of detoxification working perfectly while providing the other positive benefits of exercise. **Read on to learn a yoga routine you can do during pregnancy.**

The Natural Pregnancy Handbook

• •

The Phases of Pregnancy

The way women experience pregnancy is as varied as women themselves, says Kate Koyote, midwife and co-founder of the Matraea midwifery practice, alternative health centre, and line of organic teas, herbal balms, and birth kits. Her midwifery practice does about 50 percent of births in the Cowichan Valley of British Columbia. She herself has five children, and each pregnancy was also varied. When she first meets with pregnant women, they come with all sorts of emotions that range from excited to scared, or the woman may be laid-back and her partner extremely anxious. During the first visits, Koyote works with her clients to make sure they understand the midwifery model of care, which is based on being the woman's partner in creating a healthy pregnancy and birth, as well as establishing how they are feeling both mentally and physically. Women who work with midwives in Canada usually have more access to and longer visits with their care provider, and in most provinces, such as B.C., they also have a choice about where they want to birth, whether at home or in a hospital.

Pre-Embryonic Phase (First Two Weeks)

Pregnancy begins with conception when that lucky sperm and its corresponding genetic *and epigenetic* material unites with the woman's egg and her genetic and epigenetic material and begins its journey of great influence inside the environment of the mother. Most women are as unaware of the moment of conception as they are of all the other cellular events that make up life. The first two weeks are a time of rapid cell division as the embryo-to-be moves from the fallopian tube, where fertilization generally occurs, to the uterus, where the growing cluster of cells implants into the uterine lining around day ten. By the end of the first two weeks, the placenta has begun forming, and levels of Early Pregnancy Factor, an immunosuppressant protein, is already being manufactured.

First Trimester (Embryonic Phase)

The overwhelming experience for most pregnant women during the first trimester is one of nausea, vomiting, and lack of appetite, which affects 60 to 75 percent of pregnant women the world over. Indeed, it seems to transcend race, ethnicity, region, class, and lifestyle. It also transcends the morning and can affect women day and night, and while it often passes with the first trimester, sometimes it doesn't (as I discovered in my second pregnancy). The other common experience in the first trimester is fatigue. Elevated levels of progesterone are one of the culprits. Progesterone helps build up the uterine lining and slightly suppress the mother's immune response so that her body doesn't fight off the baby as a foreign invader (having suffered from parasites, I can confirm there is nothing as similar to that experience as the first trimester of pregnancy). The progesterone, combined with the relaxin (which helps relax the joints and widen the pelvis), work together to slow digestion, so that your body has the most opportunity to get nutrients out of food.

If you have just read the last chapter on nutrition, you may be cursing my name as you struggle to eat *anything*, let alone *everything* important for growing that baby. For most women, including myself, eating everything supposedly necessary was impossible. If this is the case for you, focus on bone broths, lightly-steeped pregnancy teas (such as from ginger or red raspberry leaf), and try your best to get your cod liver oil and folate supplements down to aid in the massive brain development during this time. Your body will likely guide you in avoiding many airborne toxins and even alcohol, coffee, and that kind of thing, which so many pregnant women report make them feel nauseated in their first trimester that a number of my friends say this is how they knew they were pregnant. As well, work your best to avoid junk food, indoor air pollution, and skincare pollutants. Indeed, because I more than once stopped to vomit while passing a leaf blower or when opening a new bottle of skin cream, I am convinced that the purpose of morning sickness is in part to help us avoid the very toxins to which we are most vulnerable, especially during this early period. Unfortunately, it also makes it hard to stomach that prenatal vitamin and liver. Koyote, the midwife, says that she counsels her patients that if they just can't stomach their prenatal vitamin, to skip it during this period because it's more important to focus on food sources of nutrition, stay hydrated, and avoid potential toxins. Most women want to avoid pharmaceutical medicines for morning sickness, and she encourages her patients to try all of the natural options first, including acupuncture and acupressure, ginger, herbal teas, and B vitamins. (See the next section for more ideas.) As well, eating protein-rich snacks at regular intervals can help keep the blood sugar stabilized, which can also prevent nausea.

Weeks Three Through Seven

During this period, the baby-to-be is called an embryo and begins to develop all of its essential parts and organs: the heart begins to beat, the head and brain begin to form, and the baby's first movements and reflexes begin. At the end of this time, the embryo looks like a miniature baby and is about half an inch long. Drug, alcohol, and toxin exposure during this period are the most correlated with

De-Stress the Thyroid

Bethany Hays, MD, has spent 34 years in obstetrics, founded a non-profit holistic healthcare centre called True North, and serves on the board of the Institute for Functional Medicine. Hays also knows a lot about the importance of the thyroid gland. She lost her own thyroid as a young woman between her first and second babies when she developed cancer that was likely caused by childhood irradiation.

The thyroid gland, which sits near the neck, is responsible for energy production and metabolism of all the cells in the body, including the brain. It works closely with the adrenal glands, found near the kidneys, on issues related to hormones, using and conserving energy, and the stress response. If the adrenals are under chronic stress — from daily life, diet, or environmental factors — they will tell the thyroid to slow down to help keep from over-drawing the adrenal bank account. Numerous environmental toxins directly affect the thyroid, as well, including most of the POPs (PERC, dioxins, PCBs, chemical flame retardants, and PFOAs), heavy metals, pesticides, plastics, soy, and fluoride. "Thyroid is the sentinel gland for the environment," says Hays.

All of these stresses can lead to autoimmune hypothyroidism, which is responsible for the vast majority of all thyroid problems in North America. Hypothyroidism can result in fatigue, weight gain, thinning hair, digestive problems, constipation, and hormonal issues, and has even been linked to issues of the developing brain, such as developmental delays, ADHD, and autism. It is also a cause of infertility and miscarriage. "The machinery has to be very carefully balanced to create sperm [and] ova, and having thyroid far enough out of the range it is supposed to be in adds to the problems of getting those things to happen and in the right order.

"I think Mother Nature's approach is that if life is too stressful, there is no need to be making babies. If they don't, they may get pregnant, but will they stay pregnant? Does the baby's brain form normally?" If a person is able to improve their environment and reduce stress, then their thyroid will work better. Hays says that to really address the issues of the thyroid, we need to "upstream" to focus on the causes, rather than the symptoms. The tips in this chapter will help. Learn more about Dr. Hays and reducing stress in Chapter 7.

abnormalities of structure or form, such as to the shape or function of the heart, eyes, arms, legs, ears, palate, teeth, and, near the end of that time, external genitals.

Weeks 8 Through 12 to 14

During this period the baby-to-be begins to grow hair and fingernails. It is possible to determine a boy from a girl, and the embryo is able to make facial expressions and even sucking motions with the lips. The eyes are almost completely developed, but they remain closed. The baby is able to drink amniotic fluid and pee it out. Weeks 8 to 14 are particularly sensitive for the developing sperm in a baby boy.

Second Trimester (Fetal Stage)

Weeks 13 Through 27

For me, as for many women, the second trimester was the golden time of pregnancy. I was finally able to pick myself up out of bed in the morning and avoid that afternoon nap, and by the end I was even able to return to my favourite pastime of freshwater swimming. The nausea eased up, and while I was still sensitive to smells, I could again walk into the kitchen and open the dishwasher without retching. Perhaps just as rewarding during this trimester is being able to finally feel the baby growing and moving inside. As well, the changes of pregnancy are in full swing: likely your breasts have grown, your body is filling with extra fluid and blood, and a bit of extra fat is being stored all over (remember, you need that for growing the baby and creating milk, so don't worry about it as long as it is from high-quality, organic sources, in which case it will build great milk and disappear quickly).

This is likely the time of pregnancy you will be feeling the best, so it's important to eat particularly well during this period. The second trimester is the time to consume plenty of protein and calcium to aid in building the baby's muscle, skin, fingernails (from protein), skeletal system (from calcium), and brain (from fats). During the fifth and sixth months, the baby-to-be's milk teeth start to develop in the uterus. The second trimester is also a time of rapid brain growth. At every opportunity, you want to eat high-quality, fat-rich protein because your body cannot store it and the baby uses it daily. If you restrict your calories at this point, your body will use the protein you eat as fuel and rob the baby of the nutrients it needs to build muscles, skin, and fingernails. As well, eat super-clean, calcium-rich foods so that the baby does not need to rob your stores to build her bones. Calcium is more viable in fermented dairy than plain old milk (remember: organic, whole). It's also in leafy greens, legumes, and seafood. You may find that you benefit tremendously during this time from frequent fat- and protein-rich snacks in order to maintain healthy blood sugar levels.

Many women also return to an exercise program. Gentle exercise such as yoga and water aerobics can be low impact and protect the joints. Women who are more physically active need to be aware of their changing centres of gravity and their bodies' different needs. Koyote says this is also when she starts discussing gestational diabetes with her clients. The treatment of gestational diabetes is diet and exercise, and thus prevention is the same. Pregnancy itself is considered a bit of a diabetic state because the placenta releases hormones that slow down the sugar to direct it through the mother and into the baby. The fundal height measurements — the measurement between the pubic bone and the belly button — is one indicator at this point that the baby's development is progressing normally. Typically the fundal height measurement equals the number of weeks pregnant.

Because of the importance of protein during the second trimester, particular attention should be given to finding sources that are of the highest quality possible and to avoiding soy, which has been shown to be able to affect the developing hormone system and sex organs of the baby-to-be.

Third Trimester (Fetal Stage)

Week 27 to the End of Pregnancy

I found the beginning of the third trimester a relief because I could regularly feel the baby move and I knew that the baby could survive if born early. By the end of the third trimester, the magic of pregnancy had worn off. My first baby was nearly two weeks past her due date — which, while being totally normal, was causing me a great deal of anticipation. I had gotten the room ready, folded all the baby clothes, and set up the birthing tub. I could barely sleep. Nothing was comfortable. My belly was enormous: it felt like a creature all its own. As well, by this time, my emotions were running high, and if I got particularly upset, my nose would spring a bloody leak: the blood vessels in the nose expand during pregnancy and that, with the increased blood supply, puts more pressure on those delicate vessels. In terms of appetite and brain fog, it felt like the first trimester all over again. Indeed, the pregnant body and brain are flooded with hormones, in particular estrogen and progesterone, and a mother-to-be can be more irritable, weepy, and anxious than she would be otherwise.

As a midwife, Koyote says that in this trimester she encourages women to focus on the positioning of the baby. By about 32 to 34 weeks, the baby is of the size and weight that positioning makes a difference. Optimal fetal positioning is the concept of getting the baby positioned for ease of birth, which means having the baby's head down and facing the spine of the mother, with chin tucked. Ideally, the baby's back will be on the mother's left. When the baby is in this position, the natural shape of the pelvis helps the baby wind its way out with the crown of the baby's head, which is the smallest part, in the lead. This helps to prevent back labour, which is when the baby's back is to the mother's back, a situation that can increase the duration of labour and the chance of a C-section being required. If women focus on their posture — not letting the curve of their back get too

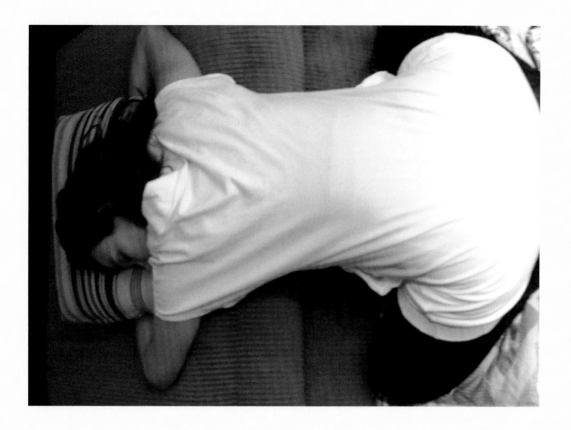

exaggerated and their bellies pulling forward and down — and their position while sitting, driving, and lying, they can help encourage optimal fetal positioning. When a pregnant mom sits on a couch with her feet up, her pelvis becomes a hammock and the baby will lie with his back in the curve of that hammock. That's the opposite of what's ideal. The heaviest parts of the baby — the crown of the head laterally or the back horizontally — will naturally want to move to the bottom. To use gravity to your advantage, sit on the couch sideways and lean forward a bit on the armrest, put a rolled-up towel under your sitting bones while driving a car, and lie on your left side at night. As well, exercises where you are on all fours — knees and hands — and gently tilt your pelvis, or where you lie across or sit on a large exercise ball, can help with ideal positioning.

This trimester is also when Koyote speaks with her clients about the benefits of perineal massage. "It's really a perineal stretch," says Koyote. "For a lot of women, the fear of childbirth is the fear of tearing," and gently stretching and preparing the perineum can help. "You will never do a stretch that will feel as intense as when you have the actual baby," she says, but perineal massage creates a body memory so that in the moment of birth a woman is more able to breathe into the stretch and relax.

By the end of the third trimester, fluid and blood volume have expanded signifi-cantly, and there is a naturally occurring anemia at this point. Koyote likes to check iron and hemoglobin levels at this time to ensure it stays in the normal range. She also recommends taking herbal teas with red raspberry leaf and nettle, traditional herbs used throughout time for uterus toning and support. They can also help with anemia. "If you were going to sign yourself up for the Boston marathon, you would train. You wouldn't just sign up and then go the next day. The uterus is the same thing." Braxton Hicks contractions are one way the uterus practises for its big work, and those will also often start by the end of the third trimester.

The third trimester for the baby is one of continued rapid brain development, with the weight of the brain tripling. The rapid development means more vulnerability to drugs, nutritional deficits, and toxins. It's a great time to keep eating that protein and essential fatty acids, especially from fish and fish oils.

Natural Pregnancy Remedies for Common Concerns

Need I even say it? Home remedies are not the same as having a midwife or medical professional who knows you, your body, and your growing baby-to-be. The home remedies below are merely a sample of recipes and old wives' cures, some used for many hundreds of years, to help get women and baby safely and comfortably through pregnancy. The aromatherapy suggestions are made with the guidance of aromatherapist Heather Gibson and the homeopathy suggestions are thanks to classical homeopath Sonya MacLeod. You can learn more about them in the sidebars in this section. There is a wealth of information out there to help you on your journey to becoming the expert on caring for yourself and your growing baby; some of it is listed in the resource section at the end of the book. Becoming that expert means becoming a better observer of your own needs as well as your baby's and knowing when you need more help. A good healthcare provider will be your partner in helping find natural remedies where appropriate and helping you determine when more emergency intervention is needed. Dr. Aviva Romm — medical doctor, midwife, herbalist, and author — says this about using herbs in pregnancy: "Overall, most herbs have a high safety profile with little evidence of harm. Pregnant [mamas] commonly experience minor symptoms and discomforts for which the use of natural remedies may be gentler and safer than over-the-counter and prescription pharmaceuticals."

Remember, the remedies below are a guideline only, and while homeopathy, particularly the kind taken as "sugar pills," is unlikely to cause direct harm, herbal remedies can be more potent and should be used with caution and guidance during pregnancy. There are some herbs better not consumed internally at all during pregnancy, according to Romm: these include the abortificants (tansy, safflower, rue, mugwort, yarrow, scotch broom, angelica, wormwood, and pennyroyal), stimulating laxatives (castor oil, buckthorn, and aloes), phytoestrogens (hops, isoflavone extracts, and red clover), and other herbs such as comfrey, borage, barberry, goldenseal, and Oregon grape. If you are in an acute situation of any kind during pregnancy — such as a prolonged headache, extreme dehydration, or severe swelling — these are signs that you need to seek immediate medical help from a professional.

Herbal Pregnancy Tea Recipe

Red raspberry leaf is the herb for pregnancy: it can help calm first trimester symptoms like nausea and third trimester symptoms like anemia. It's mineral-rich and helps tone the uterus. Other herbs that are generally agreed to be safe for use as tea in pregnancy include mint, chamomile, lemon balm, nettles, rose hips, ginger, and small amounts of echinacea to treat cold symptoms. Always use organic herbs to minimize pesticide exposures.

Ingredients:
2 tablespoons organic, dried red raspberry leaf (*uterine tonic that provides vitamins A, B, C, and E, and calcium, iron, and potassium; also helpful for increasing fertility in men and women*)
1 tablespoon organic, dried nettle leaves (*uterine tonic that provides vitamins A, C, D, and K, and calcium and potassium*)
  You can also add any one or a combination of the following:

  - 2 teaspoons lemon balm to support nervous system, digestion, and provide iron, calcium, and potassium
  - 2 teaspoons oat straw to nourish nervous system and provide vitamins A, C, E, and B, and calcium, zinc, iron, and magnesium
  - 2 teaspoons rose hips to add flavour and vitamin C
  - 2 teaspoons mint to add flavour and enhance digestion (**Caution:** used postpartum, mint can reduce production of breast milk)
  - 2 teaspoons chamomile for relaxation and to enhance sleep
  - 1 teaspoon shaved ginger can help in the first trimester with nausea (if you can stomach it)

Directions:
Use 1 tablespoon of the mixed tea leaves of your choice (see above) per 2 cups (500ml) of boiling water. Steep for 20 to 30 minutes, strain, and then discard the herbs. Drink a cup 2 to 3 times a day.

Morning Sickness

In the section on nutrition I talked about the importance of magnesium. Another one of the things magnesium does is help balance blood sugar. Extreme highs and lows are part of what causes morning sickness. Pregnancy hormones can interfere with the absorption of magnesium, and since 80 percent of people are already magnesium deficient, you probably need more. I recommend using a magnesium spray: it's effectively absorbed through the skin, and you can take it this way even when you are too sick to stomach it. The first few times you use it, it can sting a bit, but that quickly passes as you get used to it. Magnesium deficiency can also cause body odour, so try using your spray on your armpits, where it's readily absorbed and can be part of a healthier deodorizing option than conventional deodorants. Other sources include magnesium supplements and magnesium drinks such as Natural Calm. Because our soils have become increasingly depleted in magnesium, it's nearly impossible to get enough through food alone, but eating seeds and nuts can also help.

Other natural morning sickness cures include vitamin B6 (typically three doses of 25 mg three times a day), or, for greater effect, vitamin B injections under the care of a naturopath or physician. Ginger has also been shown to be effective and safe during pregnancy. Try ginger candies or homemade naturally fermented ginger beer (see page 67 in the **Green Eating Recipe Handbook**). I also enjoyed and found relief from homemade bone broth, which can be made with the addition of ginger and nutritional yeast to make it a source of all of Grandma's nutritional cures at once, although for truly bad cases of nausea, it might be wise to do additional supplementation, as well.

Acupuncture and acupressure can help relieve the nausea of pregnancy. You can work with a TCM to receive acupuncture or use acupressure at home. I used acupressure bands to help my morning sickness. These are also sold as motion sickness bands and are meant to be worn so that they press against the acupressure point just a finger's width above the inside of the wrist.

Homeopathy can help, as well, with the most common remedy being Nux Vomica 30c taken two to three times a day. Aromatherapy may also help, so try a drop of ginger essential oil on the palms of your hands and inhale. Or put a few drops of pure essential oils with citrus scents like orange or lemon on a bandana or scarf around your neck, or put a few in a vaporizer or in some water on the stove. Citrus scents can also help with fatigue; put a few drops on your hands and inhale and massage on the back of your neck.

Varicose Veins

The blood volume increases during pregnancy, and increased progesterone can cause varicose veins, which commonly appear in the legs, but can also appear as hemorrhoids or vulvar varicosities, when blood pools inside the pelvic veins deeper inside the body. The good news is that all forms of varicose veins typically diminish or disappear in the year after birth. The bad news is that they can become more likely in subsequent pregnancies. During pregnancy you can help prevent them by eating a healthy diet with plentiful good fats and by avoiding foods that promote constipation, such as refined flour, sugar, and processed foods. As well, avoid wearing high heels and sitting or standing in the same position — especially crossing your legs while sitting — for long periods. Natural treatment options include chiropractic and acupuncture care to help with circulation and the general health of the pelvic area and nerves. It can also help to partake in gentle exercise, wear maternity support hose, sleep on your left side to relieve pressure on the inferior vena cava, drink plenty of water, and elevate your legs (see the Legs up the Wall pose instructions on page 177 in the **Prenatal Yoga Handbook**). Try drinking pregnancy herbal teas with nettle leaf or oat straw. The homeopathic remedies that can help include Hamamelis for varicose veins and Sepia for hemorrhoids; both can be safely used during pregnancy in the potency of 30c two to three times a day. Witch hazel compresses (see below) can help with varicose veins in the anus and vulva area.

How to Make Witch Hazel Compresses

Witch hazel has anti-inflammatory properties and is a natural antibacterial. Pour 1 to 2 tablespoons (15–30ml) on a reusable menstrual pad and freeze it before using to help ease pain associated with vulvar varicoses, hemorrhoids, or healing after giving birth.

Swelling, High Blood Pressure, and Preeclampsia Prevention

Preeclampsia is a serious medical condition and the second leading cause of maternal death in the U.S. It's marked by sudden and severe swelling, hypertension, and protein in the urine, and it typically occurs in late pregnancy. Swelling in itself is uncomfortable at best.

Obstetrician Tom Brewer established a link between preeclampsia and protein deficiency in the 1970s. **The Brewer Diet** is based on preventing the ravages of preeclampsia by eating 100 grams of high-quality protein from meat, poultry, fish, eggs, and milk. That's four or five small servings of meat or fish every day. A can of wild salmon is two servings that equal 45 grams of total protein, 100 grams of steak or chicken breast both have about 20 grams, an egg yolk has 12 grams, a glass of whole milk has 8 grams, and just ten almonds has 2.5 grams. You can further enhance this diet by avoiding fried and processed foods and increasing your potassium, calcium, and magnesium levels.

Meditative practices, gentle exercise, fresh air, and anything that helps reduce stress — even reading — can help prevent high blood pressure. And the discomfort of swelling is further helped by getting the legs or arms above the heart. The most common homeopathic remedy prescribed to bring down swelling and edema is Apis 30c taken two to three times a day.

Avoiding Gestational Diabetes

Gestational diabetes affects up to 9 percent of pregnant women, and while its symptoms usually disappear soon after giving birth, both mother and child are at greater risk of developing Type 2 diabetes. Researchers have been using the data from the Nurses' Health Study, the same one that has given so much information on fertility and diet, and followed more than 6,000 women to understand why gestational diabetes is such a strong indicator of future diabetes. The conclusion is that epigenetics play a role and that environmental factors are turning on and off genes that make diabetes more likely. For instance, researchers found that drinking soda was more likely to flip the switch for the obesity gene. While much is left to be studied, gestational diabetes is an early indicator that environmental factors such as diet, sleep, and stress have already begun to affect you and your child. It also means that you might be predisposed to gestational diabetes through no fault of your own.

Prevention in this case is the same as the cure: better diet and exercise. In particular, the advice of nutritionist Margaret Floyd Barry is relevant: always consume carbohydrates with a healthy, fatty protein; skip refined sugars and carbohydrates; front load your day and your meals with those good fatty proteins; and partake in gentle exercise. As well, try sipping on a mix of apple cider vinegar with water before meals. Vitamin D, in conjunction with vitamins A and K, can also be helpful in preventing gestational diabetes. Anti-inflammatory foods like omega-3 oils, olive oil, fatty fish, and leafy greens can help, and so can reducing stress and getting at least eight hours of sleep. If you develop full-blown gestational diabetes, then what might be fine in other pregnancies — such as eating a piece of cake every so often or starting the day with a bowl of cereal — can put you and your baby at risk because, in short, your body and the baby's body while inside you can't handle sugars, including simple carbohydrates, even the natural kind. Besides diet and lifestyle changes, homeopathic phosphoric acid can be tried at 30c two to three times a day.

Heartburn Help

Heartburn is common in later pregnancy and is caused by the pressure the growing uterus puts on the digestive system and the relaxation of the esophageal sphincter

Inspiring Mamas:
Adopting Aromatherapy for Families

Heather Gibson is a clinical aromatherapist and a mother extraordinaire: she also has three biological children and four adopted children, and she has fostered more than 20 kids. Gibson has turned to aromatherapy to help her manage her own health as well as many of the more difficult behavioural issues that she encounters as a parent. Gibson has used aromatherapy clinically to help clients relax during therapy. "It's a tool, not a cure-all," she says about using essential oils for health.

Essential oils can be used topically as a cosmetic or breathed in as aromatherapy, or some can even be taken internally. "Aromatic use is the safest way to use essentials oils and also the best way to use them for the emotions," says Gibson. "It goes straight to your limbic system and affects you more powerfully." She cautions that not all essential oils are made the same, and there isn't true oversight of essential oil claims such as "pure." When looking for a good brand, be wary of grocery store brands, many of which aren't pure and can even have added petroleum by-products or fragrance oils. You can learn more about aromatherapy and essential oils for pregnancy and parenting at Gibson's website www.MyHealthEmpowered.com and try many of her recommendations in this section.

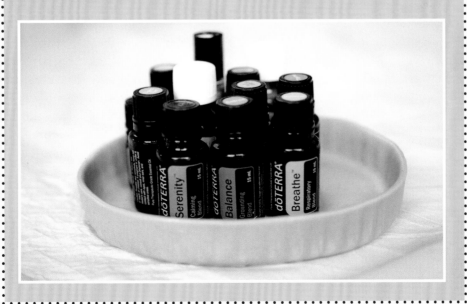

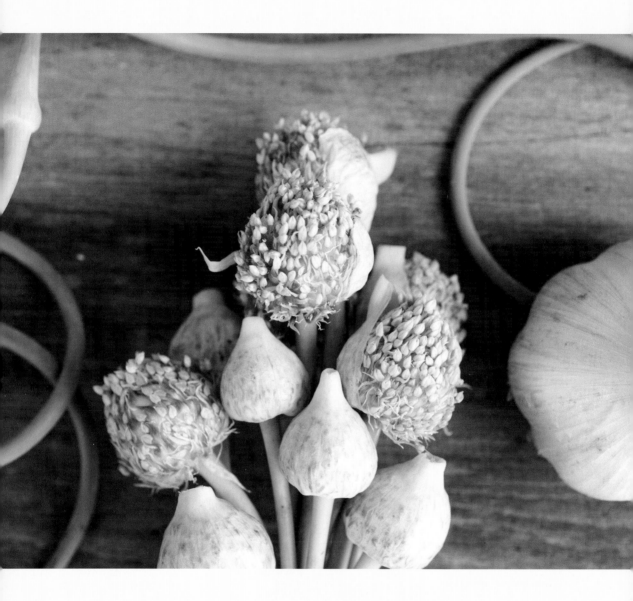

by the rise in progesterone. The midwives at Matraea recommend watermelon (if you like it) and almonds, and eating small meals, not eating right before bed, and propping yourself up on pillows in bed. Aromatherapy can also help: try peppermint essential oil or a mix of equal amounts of lemon, mandarin, and sweet orange essential oil. Put a few drops of either blend on a tissue or on a scarf that you wear around your head. Or mix a few drops with an edible oil (such as olive or sesame oil) and use it on your chest. The homeopathic remedy Pulsatilla 30c, in two to three doses a day, can help a woman who has heartburn as well as other symptoms of indigestion during pregnancy.

Ease Those Leg Cramps

I was prone to leg and foot cramps, otherwise known as charley horses, in my pregnancy. Yikes! I found that a diet rich in magnesium, yoga stretches, and flexing the leg during the cramp could all help. You can also try a warm bath with half a cup of Epsom salts with essential oils added: 3 drops geranium, 10 drops lavender, and 2 drops cypress.

Treating Yeast Infections with Garlic

Vaginal yeast infections can be more common during pregnancy, perhaps because of fluctuating hormones. And while you don't have to worry about the infection hurting the baby, if you still have it during labour, the baby may be more likely to develop thrush. Vaginal application of garlic is a cure I have used myself for treating yeast infections. Some midwives also say vaginal garlic suppositories used regularly at the end of pregnancy may be able to rid a woman of Group B strep (GBS).

Take a clove of garlic and peel it, being very careful not to nick the clove. Wrap the clove in a small rectangle of clean gauze and then tie closed the ends with a bit of equally clean, thin string, leaving a tail. In the end, the whole thing ought to look like a DIY tampon. Dip the cloth into organic, food-grade olive oil or coconut oil to help with insertion. Insert into the vagina and leave in overnight. Expect a bit of discharge. Change every twelve hours and use for three to five days. If the infection is more advanced, then you can purposely create a small nick in the garlic, or even cut the clove in half, significantly increasing your exposure to the garlic's antibacterial and antifungal properties. Beware: this increased exposure comes with quite a sting.

Treating Headaches in Pregnancy

Headaches can occur during pregnancy for a variety of reasons, including low blood sugar, stress, and hormonal changes, as well as all the regular headache triggers, such as not getting enough water or suffering from constipation. If headaches during pregnancy are frequent or more intense than usual, talk with your doctor or midwife, because they can be a sign of much more serious problems, such as the onset of preeclampsia. For routine headache, tea may help. See the recipe that follows. Aromatherapy using lavender, lemon, peppermint, spearmint, sweet orange, or tea tree oil might help, as may acupressure. There is a pressure point on the hand in the fleshy part between the thumb and the pointer finger; if you try probing around in there, you will often find a more sensitive spot. Press on this with the thumb and forefinger of your other hand for as long as possible.

Inspiring Mamas:
Homeopathy to the Rescue

Sonya McLeod, B.A., DCH, R.Hom., found her way to studying homeopathy after she had her second daughter and found herself plagued by health problems with which her doctors couldn't help.

Classical homeopathy originated in Germany more than 200 years ago, and it is based on the idea that the body can be taught to heal itself and works on the energetic level. To do this, homeopathic doctors operate under the principle that "like cures like." To make homeopathic remedies, they use nano amounts of a natural material — such as a mineral or a plant or, say, a bit of bee — and dilute it many times. In homeopathy, the more diluted something is, the stronger it is. For example, a homeopathic remedy given to a person suffering from insomnia is coffea, a remedy made from coffee. The final homeopathic remedy is so dilute that there isn't more than a nanoparticle of the original substance, in this case coffee, left within. Rather, an energetic imprint has been made on the substance in which it is diluted — such as sugar water or alcohol — and that imprint is what stimulates the body to heal itself.

Homeopathy is so different from our usual understanding of chemistry and pharmaceutical medicines that it has garnered very vocal skeptics — from medical doctors to journalists — who say it isn't conceivable that homeopathy works. Nevertheless, in many places, such as England, France, Switzerland, Italy, the Netherlands, and India, it is so popular that it has been incorporated into mainstream medicine. It's called the leading "alternative" treatment used by physicians in Europe. At the very least, what skeptics and homeopaths alike agree upon is that homeopathy is so gentle that it is virtually impossible to cause harm from its use.

McLeod recommends that pregnant women look into cell salts — very gentle, mineral-based homeopathic remedies — which can be used to help balance or provide minerals during key times of pregnancy. To learn more about cell salts and what remedies might be an addition to your pregnancy, visit a homeopath or try out McLeod's website at www.littlemountainhomeopathy.com, or try some of her general recommendations in this section. McLeod cautions, "If after a few doses there is no improvement, a person is advised to move on to another remedy or seek the help of a trained homeopath."

Headache Tea Recipe

Ingredients:
1/2 cup dried lemon balm leaves
1/2 cup nettles
1/2 cup rose hips
1/2 cup spearmint leaves

Directions:
Use 1 teaspoon of tea leaves per 2 cups (500ml) of boiling water. Steep for 20 to 30 minutes, strain, and discard the herbs. Drink a cup 2 to 3 times a day.

Moodiness and Depression

There is a lot going on during pregnancy and after, as hormones surge through the body and life changes unalterably for most women. Nutrition can help prevent some of the moodiness and mild depression that can come with pregnancy. There are a number of studies linking adequate intake of DHA, especially from fish oils, to lower rates of postpartum depression. Additional nutritional support may be necessary if you have already improved your diet but moodiness and depression continue, or if they are severe. Extreme fatigue in pregnancy can be a sign of certain nutritional deficits, especially vitamin B12 and iron, and may warrant further testing.

For common moodiness or mild depression associated with normal pregnancy, homeopathy might help. Pulsatilla is for women who are very weepy, sentimental, and all over the place emotionally during pregnancy. Ignatia is good if the predominate emotion is grief, such as from losses in the past or lots of fear. For postpartum depression, Sepia is recommended. Take 30c two to three times a day.

Stretch Mark Prevention

It's not really possible to cure stretch marks, only to reduce their appearance and try to prevent them. You will know if you are more susceptible if you already have stretch marks from a previous pregnancy or growth spurt. Fortunately, genetics or having previous stretch marks does not mean you can't try to prevent future stretch marks, and diet is the key. Stretch marks are actually a tearing of the tissue in the dermis or middle layer of the skin that occurs when it is stretched beyond its capacity. That capacity can be somewhat increased through diet. Great foods that help include gelatin, which you can get through high-quality, natural supplements or by eating that ever-so-wonderful home-made bone broth (consider adding chicken feet for extra gelatin). Fish oil is another great food supplement that is high in vitamin A and anti-inflammatory omega-3 oils and can help with elasticity. Butter, olive oil, and coconut oil can also help with this. Eat antioxidant-rich fruits and vegetables, especially those high in vitamin C, which helps make the collagen necessary for skin elasticity. Foods rich in vitamins A, E, K, and B-complex will also help with the suppleness of the skin. The good news about preventing stretch marks through diet is that these same foods will help the perineum to stay soft and supple, thus making tearing during birth less likely. Skin-based prevention for stretch marks is not likely enough on its own because it is the middle layer of the skin where the tearing occurs, but nevertheless, having skin that feels rich and hydrated at the very least helps prevent the discomfort of growing larger and the itchy-dry skin feeling that may accompany it. Try the belly balm that follows for stretch marks. As well, you can try homeopathic Calc Fluor 6X cell salts one to two times per day.

Blossoming Belly Balm

Most apothecaries I work with recommend a base of cocoa butter and coconut oil. I personally find coconut oil a bit drying, so I will often supplement with unrefined sesame oil or olive oil, which can make the final product a bit runnier, but I like the feel. Try using two parts cocoa butter to one part other oil. Experiment to find your favourite!

Then add other oils for additional nourishment, such as rose hip oil, vitamin E oil, or sweet almond oil. Try any of these at about 1⁄2 part ratio to the oil. See the recipe below for clarification.

Ingredients:
1⁄2 cup (109g) cocoa butter
1⁄4 cup (52g) coconut oil
2 tablespoons (30ml) rose hip seed oil, vitamin E oil, and/or sweet almond oil
5–10 drops lavender essential oil
5–10 drops helichrysum essential oil
5–10 drops of myrrh

Directions:
Warm cocoa butter and coconut (or other) oil in a double boiler until both are melted. Then add the rose hip seed oil, vitamin E oil, and/or sweet almond oil. Stir. Remove from heat. Add essential oils. Pour into jar. Apply regularly.

Labour Help

There are a lot of old wives' tales about how best to bring on labour. Most midwives, however, will caution that the baby will come when the time is right.

That being said, the information on proper positioning and gentle exercise leading up to the birth can help with a speedier labour. Perineal massage, water birth, and diets rich in omega-3 fatty acids, fish oils, and vitamins A, E, K, and B-complex will help to avoid tearing. Taking adequate amounts of fish oils can help soften the perineum. And drinking pregnancy tea with red raspberry leaves can help prepare the uterus.

Homeopathy offers a few helpers as well, including Pulsatilla 30c to turn a breech baby and Caulophyllum and Cimicifuga 30c. The latter two can be alternated (one in the morning, one in the evening) for overdue labours, and for a non-progessive labour alternate 200c potency of Caulophyllum with Cimicifuga every half hour or so. (Never take Cimicifuga or Caulophyllum during the first or second trimesters.) And for panicked fathers or grandparents during labour, a dose or two of Aconitum 200c will help. Arnica 30c pellets can help with healing and bruising after the labour.

Aromatherapy can help a person relax more into the labour. Try any of these out beforehand to find your favourite: lavender, wild orange, and peppermint, or bergamot. Use a diffuser for best results.

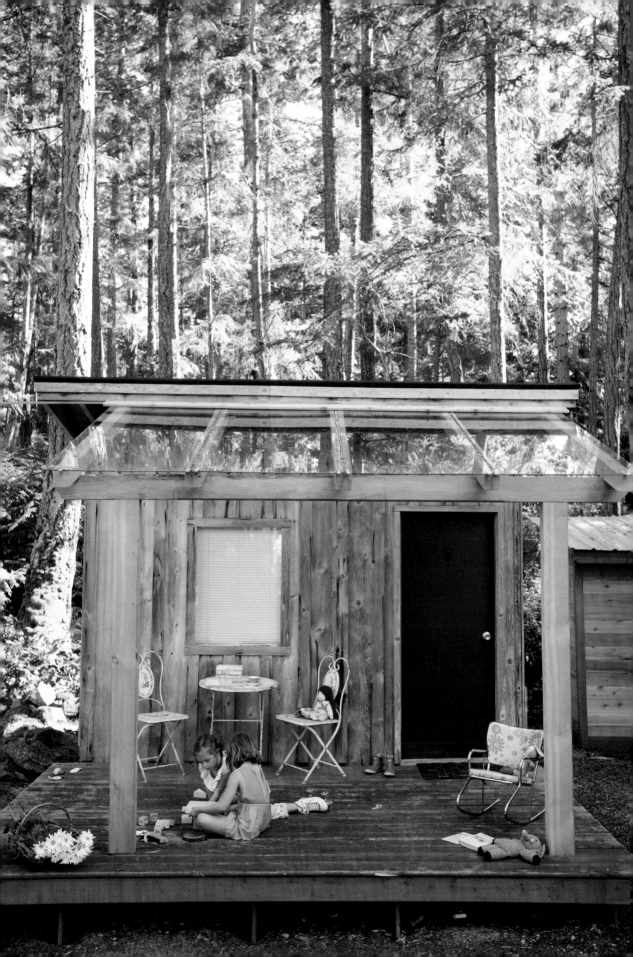

Greening
Your Home

• •

It doesn't take a lot of imagination or a lot of science to see how traces of the chemicals in our homes might end up in our kids. Living with a baby makes it all too clear. My children have finished off their breakfasts with a little chew on the table and eaten many things off the floor. My eldest has stuck her finger in the cleaning powder (luckily made with baking soda) and had window cleaner (vinegar in a bottle) sprayed in her face. My youngest has eaten a tube of toothpaste (thank goodness it was about as natural and fluoride-free as it gets), swallowed a bottle of pills (luckily, homeopathic), and swallowed a bit of candle (it was un-dyed beeswax) to further remind me of how important it is to keep everything in my house as green as possible. While these are obvious examples of the potential health hazards of the things we bring into our homes, the greatest culprits are usually invisible, or at least miniscule.

The Research

We know that fetuses are particularly vulnerable to air pollution. Indoor air is typically two to five times more polluted than the outside air, whether a person lives in the city or the country. Indoor air is a useful indicator for judging just how green many home products are, giving us further reason to rethink the cheap pressed-wood cupboards or the vinyl shower curtain or even using a dry cleaner, all of which can significantly and negatively affect our indoor air quality.

The pollutants that we breathe in enter our bodies and can enter our bloodstreams and affect pregnancy outcomes. The more polluted the air, the greater the risk of low birth weight, premature birth, asthma, and disturbed physical and brain development, including ADHD, anxiety, autism, depression, development delays, and lower IQ.

Green Tip: Before You Start Renovating

One of the first things to remember is that pregnancy is not a good time to partake in renovations. You will only increase your exposure to some of the worst toxins from solvents in paint removers, lead in old paint, and VOCs in just about every new finish and other new thing that goes into a home. If a renovation just can't be avoided, leave the house for the duration of the renovation and make sure you follow all the green advice possible, particularly on finding zero-VOC finishes. There are, however, lots of ways to green your home that are safe during pregnancy and lots of little tricks to improve the quality of the indoor air in the home you have. It is possible to release extra VOCs by increasing the temperature in a room, as higher temperatures encourage products to off-gas more. Consider doing an extra "off-gassing" of all the new paints, flooring, and furniture, but beware that the VOCs might escape into the rest of the house. To do this safely, crank up the heat for a few days and securely shut the door to the room you are off-gassing. Then, open the window and use a ventilation fan to suck all those nasty chemicals out of the house — the more time to off-gas, the better.

We know a lot about some of the most troubling indoor air pollutants, such as VOCs. In one study of VOCs, the Consumer Product Safety Commission found that, while outdoor air at sample sites contained fewer than ten of these chemical toxins, indoor air at those same locations contained an average of 150. VOC concentrations can be so high inside homes and buildings that they are able to make a person perceivably and immediately sick — this is called sick building syndrome. Improving indoor air quality can have immediate benefits as well as less tangible ones. There is even research linking better in vitro fertilization (IVF) outcomes to improvements in laboratory air quality.

Five (Fixable) Sources of Indoor Air Pollution

The main indoor air polluters fall into five categories:

1. **Outdoor pollutants** can get inside on feet or through vents (think lead from our urban soils, arsenic from treated wood, or pesticides from outdoor spraying).
2. **By-products of combustion**, including polycyclic aromatic hydrocarbons (PAHs), carbon monoxide, and formaldehyde, come from vehicle exhaust, leaky furnaces, or second-hand cigarette smoke.

3. **Mould and mildew**, which can develop if drywall, paper, or wood becomes moist and doesn't dry out within 48 hours. Mould colonies release spores that can cause allergies and respiratory problems, and some are toxic.

4. **Building materials, furniture, and finishes** are often the biggest polluters in homes, and they are the ones we have the most control over. These include paint, wallpaper, carpets, furniture, pressed wood, glues, PVC products, flame-retardant fabrics and foams, and electrical items.

5. **Household cleaning products and other chemicals** have made it such that the area around the cabinet where cleaning products are stored is substantially more polluted than the rest of the air in the home. These chemicals are also a major source of childhood poisonings. There are currently 17,000 different petrochemicals available for use in the home.

In one small but fabulously specific study, the researchers correlated exposure to VOCs prenatally and in infancy from typical home renovations to an increased risk of upper respiratory disease, in particular wheezing. The strongest association was found with floor coverings of wall-to-wall carpet, PVC material, and laminate flooring and prenatal exposure. A similar study showed that children whose mothers had higher chemical burdens from household chemical products had a greater chance of developing asthma and were twice as likely to wheeze persistently throughout childhood. Yet another study specifically looking at formaldehyde exposure and its relationship to low birth weight showed the greatest correlation when exposure took place during the first trimester. Chemical flame retardants enter the air and dust of a home from couches, beds, curtains, baby car seats, and other cushioned or fabric items. Exposures to one of these chemicals, PBDEs (a chemical flame retardant), in vitro and during infancy were correlated to a 4.5-point drop in IQ and greater hyperactivity in five-year-olds.

The Sixth Fixable Polluter: Electromagnetic Fields

I can relate to really not wanting to believe that something as pervasive, and *invisible*, as electromagnetic fields (EMFs) can cause harm. Natural EMFs have been with us for thousands of years in the form of earthly and cosmic electricity and magnetism. It is only in the past one hundred years that we have seen the invention and emergence of man-made EMFs from radio frequencies, electric power lines, and x-rays. Although health issues were studied and noted, it was really after 1998, and especially after 2005, that EMFs started to become a common health concern and the term "electro-hypersensitivity" came into the vernacular.

What promoted this change? It was the incorporation of digital (computer) technologies *with* radio frequency technologies. In a few short years we saw the rapid emergence of digital cellphone technologies, Wi-Fi, DECT cordless phones, wireless baby monitors, the smart phone, smart meters, and devices that interfere with the electrical grid, such as dimmer light switches and compact fluorescent light bulbs (CFLs).

Though generally thought to be safe, there are some studies that link EMFs to possible health effects such as ADHD, brain tumours, insomnia, implantation issues in women, increased heart rate, infertility in men, leukemia, miscarriage, reduced brain function, and issues in offspring, including asthma and neurological disturbances. EMFs have been listed as a potential carcinogenic by the International Agency for Research on Cancer (IARC). Many countries in the EU have issued warnings about the effects of EMFs on children, infants, and pregnant women. Indeed, a number of the doctors that I spoke with for this book said that the rise in background levels of EMF radiation more closely matches the rise in neurological changes in children than any other curve of known neurotoxins. In the last ten years, the levels of EMF from Wi-Fi and cellphone sources have risen from negligible to exceeding precautionary levels as recommended by *The Bio-Initiative Report 2012* and the International Institute for Building-Biology & Ecology.

There have been a number of recent studies looking at the relationship of prenatal exposure and health outcomes. These studies each give us a little bit of the whole picture. They suggest that when laptops are used on the laps of pregnant women, they create electric currents in the fetus above levels known to be able to cause adverse health effects, including tumours. Animal studies show a relationship between in vitro EMF exposure and effects in the brain and kidneys. A particularly long and compelling study found that children born to women with higher EMF exposures were more than three times as likely to develop asthma. For this study they followed more than 800 Californian women and their offspring for 13 years. The research also suggests that children may absorb more EMFs than adults, just like children absorb more of the most tangible toxins — such as lead — than adults do. There are a number of ways to protect you and your children from the possible effects of EMFs. The measurement I keep in my head is that, for most sources, the effect is minimal after a three or four feet distance. Keep reading for more tangible action steps.

The Good News

There is good news in the answer to the question of what is polluting our indoor air. That's because most of the big polluters are things we can do something about. This pollution most often comes from things we bring into the house ourselves, such as furniture, stinky cleaning supplies, paints, and new baby items. Pollution also gets tracked in on our shoes, is sucked in the door from an attached garage, or wafts in through an air intake, which is particularly problematic if that air intake is near a busy road or somewhere that smokers hang out. Energy-efficient buildings are great in many ways, but they can keep fresh air from flowing in and through a house.

How to Green the Environment of Your Home

Here are a series of action steps to green your indoor environment. These are listed a bit differently from the other "How To" sections because they are broken into type of impact, but as best as possible they are also listed from ♥♥♥ (biggest impact, and possibly more work) to ♥ (quick and easy) to help you green your home and improve your indoor air quality.

1. ♥♥♥ **Green your big-ticket items.** When most people think of green or eco buildings, they think about the big-ticket items like solar panels, electric vehicle charging stations, and energy-efficient appliances, such as front-loading washing machines. Many of these items are investments that will pay for themselves in energy savings no matter what kind of home you have, and they will help you reduce your carbon footprint. Using energy is not just expensive in the short term; it's linked with many of the worst environmental issues, from climate change to air pollution. Adding insulation, solar hot water, or programmable thermostats, or swapping out old appliances for new front-loading machines or new energy-efficient refrigerators, are among the first items to consider for green investments that can have fast returns. When you have a baby on the way, many of these green investments will pay off even faster. (I remember how I longed for a front-load washer as I did loads of cloth diapers with my first baby.)

    There are often government incentives to help with investments such as solar panels, and this technology has come a long way fast in affordability and efficacy. While these big-ticket items will give you the most bang for the buck, I would encourage you to go beyond thinking about only energy efficiency and also consider indoor air quality.

2. ♥♥ **Green the shelves, bookcases, and cabinets.** Furniture is the most significant source of formaldehyde exposure in most homes. In your living room, that means you should eye with suspicion the bookcases, cabinets, side tables, desks, and even your couch. In your bedroom, bedside tables, chests of drawers, and the bed may be off-gassing VOCs, and in a child's room cribs and change tables are the big culprits. One crib is enough to raise the VOC levels in the entire home to the point where it can significantly increase a child's chance of developing asthma. The problematic chemicals, especially VOCs, may be hiding out in the material itself (particularly in composite materials such as pressed wood or particle board), in the glues that hold it together, and in the finishes.

    Neither the Canadian nor the U.S. government regulates your household furnishings for VOCs despite increasing scientific data about their long-term health effects, including formaldehyde's known link to human cancers and many of the VOCs links to asthma. The good news about formaldehyde, as with many of the VOCs, is that while they are bad for human health, they do decrease over time. That's the nature of VOCs, which are, umm, extremely volatile. So if you buy a ten-year-old fake wood bookcase from the thrift store, you will be saving yourself both money and toxic exposure.

Inspiring Mamas: Organic Sleep

Jem Terra is a single mother to three and an accidental entrepreneur. She is the owner of inBed Organics, Canada's premier natural mattress company. She makes and distributes her truly natural (and the most affordable in the class) mattresses, pillows, and bedding from Vancouver, B.C., and at www.inBedOrganics.com.

Terra found herself in the mattress business by accident. When her son was young, he had severe allergies to dust mites and mould. She tried everything, and still the dark circles under his eyes and the fatigue and other symptoms remained. "So I took apart the futon we slept on and I found mould in it. That's when all the research started."

She was startled to discover how many babies died in their beds in First World nations. She found SIDS research that showed it was higher in third and fourth children, not first-borns. "Then I found this research done in New Zealand about toxic gases that release from the chemicals in mattresses and mix with fluids — sweat, drool, pee — and bacteria from the baby. The resulting gas was heavy and slowed down their nervous systems, and the toxic gases got worse over time with every subsequent baby." She emphasizes that moms need good beds, too: for themselves and because the "chemicals in the beds enter their bodies and then the fetus and the breast milk."

Terra remembered this hole in the market later when she ended up divorced and needing a job. She laughs: "I didn't want to put my kids into daycare, and so the only option was to start a business." The mattresses she makes are entirely natural and meet flame-retardancy standards. The latex she uses is certified organic, the wool is natural and processed without added chemicals, and the covers are made of either natural (naturally mould-resistant) hemp or certified organic cotton. "I find that when I lie down on a good mattress, when I wake up, I am replenished." She tries to give that experience to everyone she can.

Buy furniture that is made with real wood and finished with water-based, preferably edible finishes, such as those made from hemp or beeswax. Be particularly careful to avoid pressed wood (aka particle board) or other composite wood products, since they are one of the biggest polluters of VOCs. Similarly, be wary of VOC-emitting glues and finishes. Look for a third-party certifying body to help you know what you are buying. FSC certifies sustainably harvested wood, and Greenguard ensures safer levels of VOCs.

But what if your budget isn't equal to the purchase of high-quality new items? Never fear. Used is usually safer in this regard: even pressed wood releases most of its VOCs after about seven years.

3. ♥♥ **Green your mattress, baby's bed, and couch.** You can avoid excess chemicals by buying a truly natural mattress made from natural rubber, organic cotton, or wool. What you want is a mattress that is naturally flame retardant because it is made entirely from noncombustible natural materials. Since all polyurethane foam is made of petroleum and is highly flammable by nature, requiring chemical flame retardants, it's better to forego that material. It's important to note that "organic" isn't a meaningful label when applied to mattresses, so beware of claims like "made with soy foam" or "made with natural latex" or even sales reps calling a mattress "organic." Instead, make sure that you ask how the company is meeting flame-retardancy standards and ask to see the Material Safety Data Sheets. You will probably pay about twice as much for a natural mattress as you would for a conventional one, but the price difference can be far less for a baby's.

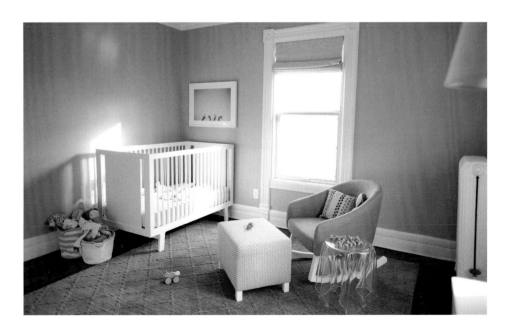

When buying a new sofa or soft chair, ideally you should look for products made from natural materials rather than polyurethane foam. Skip buying items made before 2004 or labelled "TB 117 compliant," as these are both signs that they contain chemical flame retardants. When buying new, skip the stain-guard feature, too, as it releases potentially toxic and extremely persistent perflourinated compounds. Instead, apply your own green cleaning at home or opt for steam cleaning without the use of solvents after the red wine has splashed on the white couch. If a new sofa isn't in the mix, you can sometimes do quite well with antiques that were made before the advent of polyurethane foam and chemical flame retardants. When making do with what you have, ensure that there are no cracks or tears exposing the foam innards of any of your furnishings. Mend or cover up any such fissures: duct tape to the rescue! As well, minimize time spent napping or eating on that old sofa.

4. ♥♥ **Green the carpets, flooring, window coverings, and textiles.**
Flooring is one of the primary culprits for VOC exposure in vitro, with wall-to-wall carpets being one of the worst, as they can off-gas VOCs from the material themselves and from the toxic glues used to hold them in place. And carpets, like couches and beds, collect allergens such as dust mites, mildew, and mould over time. They can also be a repository for PBDEs, bacteria, and heavy metals tracked from outside on shoes, stroller wheels, or feet. Vinyl flooring and laminate flooring were the next biggest indoor air polluters related to renovations. Both of these flooring types are made from materials that are known to release VOCs in and of themselves,

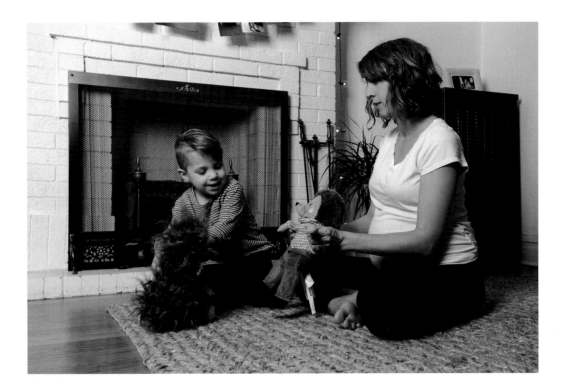

as well as relying on often toxic formaldehyde and VOC-releasing glues to hold them in place.

Healthier, greener flooring options include refinishing the wood floors that you already have (if you have them). Make sure you finish them with a low-VOC, formaldehyde-free, water-based option. New green flooring options include floors made from wood, bamboo, cork, Marmoleum, tile, and carpet tiles. If you want rugs, go with throw rugs that can be washed (by someone, at least, even if not in your home washing machine). If you do decide to go for wall-to-wall carpet, then take extra precautions to ensure it isn't placed with typical VOC-laden glues and that it is made of natural materials and pre-off-gassed in the factory.

Textiles such as permanent-press curtains are another significant source of formaldehyde in the average home. Curtains are also commonly treated with those nasty flame retardants. Window coverings such as blinds may be made with PVC that can break down over its lifetime and release phthalates into the dust and air of a home. There are a number of greener options. Curtains and other textiles made from natural materials will have far fewer VOCs, as will curtains that have been washed. Non-PVC blinds, such as those made from fabric, paper, or wood, are also a greener option.

When Money Matters More

If you are stuck with old wall-to-wall carpet that you aren't allowed to remove, consider getting throw rugs that are easier to clean to put over them. If you are going to splurge on anything, get a truly natural mattress and pillows. I haven't seen research on it (there probably isn't any), but if you can even start with a natural mattress topper over your existing futon or conventional mattress, it would mean that at least the part closest to your mouth and skin is safer. We did this to slowly build my eldest a natural mattress starting with camping mats and cotton blankets, and then graduating to an all-cotton futon, until finally we could afford a truly natural mattress.

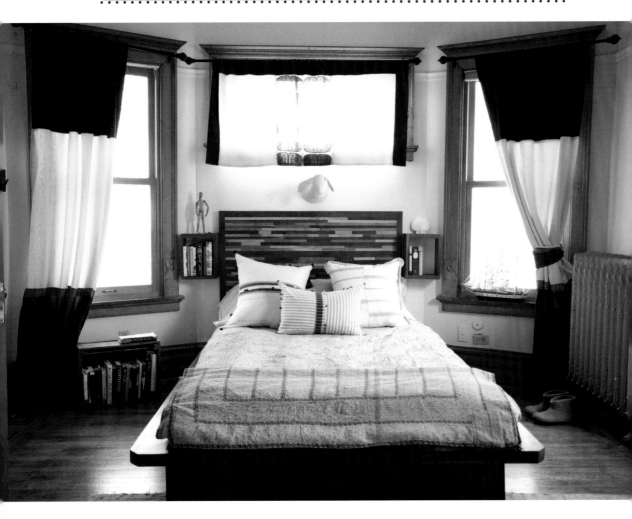

5. ♥♥ **Green the finishes, paints, and wallpaper.** The EPA says that paints and finishes are one of the top culprits in polluting our indoor air and can continue to off-gas VOCs for years after application. It is definitely ideal to forego painting while pregnant. If you can't help yourself, you'll be happy to know there are zero- and low-VOC paints available. These paints aren't without VOCs, but they have far less than typical paint: low VOC paints must have fewer than 250 g/L and zero-VOC paints fewer than 5 g/L. This means they smell better and are better for your health. You can also get paints that are so natural they are nearly edible; these include milk paint and mineral paints. I've used many of these paints in my home, and most zero-VOC paints are every bit as easy to use as typical paints. The truly VOC-free paints, such as those made from milk and minerals, are very different to work with, and the result is rich, beautiful, and more varied than typical paint. These natural paint alternatives can work great for painting wood, as well.

   Similarly, typical wallpaper is a health mess made of vinyl, adhered with VOC-laden glues, and prone to growing mould and mildew. Luckily, there are some new options that use recycled paper instead of vinyl as their base, are painted or printed with no-VOC paints, and applied with no-VOC glues. I have also used these, and since I had no previous experience with vinyl wallpaper, I found them a fun alternative, particularly if they are used just as an accent for a wall or two.

6. ♥♥ **Green cleaning and supplies.** When thinking about the worst offenders for cleaning products, you might be surprised at what can harm your health. The chemicals in dishwashing detergent, for instance, can

When Money Matters More

If your home or furniture is old or antique, then you may have lead paint. Before 1978 in the U.S. and 1980 in Canada, lead was routinely added to paint. This is only really a problem to your pregnancy if the paint is flaking, which it very well could be after almost 40 years. So get somebody (not you — you're pregnant!) to paint over it with a zero-VOC product. Yes, this is a bit more expensive, but not that much more. **Quick tip:** You can go into just about any hardware store and ask for their off-colour (didn't quite match the colour swatch) low-VOC paints and get them cheaper or even free.

be particularly harmful because the hot air vaporizes the chemicals and releases them into your home. The EPA also warns against many air fresheners that can continuously release pollutants (for example, neurotoxins and allergens) into your air. Multipurpose cleaners with added disinfectants often contain warnings about wiping down surfaces with water after the cleaner has been applied, especially if you use them on counters, cutting boards, or tables. If you are doing this, you are increasing your chances of absorbing these chemicals through your skin or along with your food.

"Bad" cleaning products are ones that pollute your indoor air quality or, even worse, are so poisonous that they are sold with skull and crossbones symbols and must be locked away for fear that a precocious child will get hold of them. You may have wondered, "How safe is it really to dump something with 'WARNING! Poison' on the label down the drain or onto the floor?" Indeed, traces of these very chemicals can end up surviving multiple water treatments and cause harm both to aquatic life and, ultimately, human life when they show up downstream in someone's water glass. Even if these chemicals make it no further than the kitchen floor, they can release toxic fumes into the air inside our homes. Besides being poisonous in concentration, they can also make us sick in dilution.

Microbes are everywhere: they make up our guts and our skin, and they surround us. We don't need to fear microbes. They aren't all bad, and microbes, such as most viruses and bacteria, can't live on dry surfaces. These microbes do like food particles, mucus, and moisture, though, so watch out for your kitchen sponge. It can be rid of most microbes by microwaving it for three minutes or boiling it in a pot of water. The hot water from your tap is not hot enough to sterilize.

Cleaning is the first defence against the spread of germs. In today's culture, we often overlook the importance of this step in our rush to go straight for the "big guns" of sanitizing or disinfecting. If a surface isn't clean, it can't effectively be sanitized. Good cleaning involves a little elbow grease and some basic ingredients like soap, water, vinegar, baking soda, microfibre cloths, and maybe an EcoLogo-certified multi-purpose cleaner. There is no proven benefit to disinfecting every surface in your home.

If you are really worried about disinfecting your home, for instance after a flu, you still must start with cleaning first. Disinfectants kill germs on a surface, and they only work if you've already removed the germ habitat. Once this is done, use the safest, least toxic, most appropriate product. White vinegar or 3 percent hydrogen peroxide applied after cleaning and left to sit for 10 minutes will kill flu viruses and salmonella. To disinfect against E. coli and listeria, heat either vinegar or hydrogen peroxide to 55°C (130°F) and leave on for a minute. Both tea tree oil and oregano oil have been found to contain antimicrobial properties. The sun also disinfects, so hang clothes to dry, open windows, and pull out those pillows for a little sun magic.

If you decide to buy a commercial cleaning product or disinfectant, read the label closely. Make sure the product lists all of its ingredients, has a meaningful third-party certification such as EcoLogo or Green Seal, and is biodegradable. Do a quick scan to verify it's free of the most harmful ingredients, such as ammonia, APEs, chlorine bleach, coal tar dyes, DEA, fragrances, sodium hydroxide, or triclosan. Companies don't have to restrict or reveal all the ingredients in cleaning products sold in North America, so extra caution should be taken. Use the sniff test: if it smells strongly of artificial fragrance or makes you sneeze or your eyes water, this is often a sign that it contains artificial fragrance to "mask" the smell of other noxious chemicals.

Making your own green cleaning products is a great option, and it can be affordable, effective, and as easy as having baking soda, vinegar, hydrogen peroxide (or another oxygen-based cleaner), microfibre cloths, and maybe a bit of lemon or tea tree oil on hand.

7. ♥♥ **Reduce your EMF exposure.** There are plenty of practical ways to reduce you and your baby-to-be's EMF exposure.

- **Ditch the big emitters** that you can live without. DECT cordless phones can usually go because they can emit even more EMFs than your cellphone. I've been really enjoying my mock 1950s payphone. ECO DECT phones that do not radiate when not in use are available in Europe, but sadly not in North America.
- **If the source of EMFs is from outside the home**, consider shielding, which involves using metallic cloth, paint, or other material to block the EMFs from entering.
- **For internet, disconnect and disable the Wi-Fi** from the router *and* the laptop. Instead, wire the devices to the router using *ethernet* cables.
- **Get your laptop and tablets off your lap and away from your body.** There is research to suggest that radiation levels this close can harm you and your developing baby. It is also beneficial to keep off your laptops and tablets at night, when they are most likely to disrupt sleep.
- **While you may not be ready to toss the cellphone, you can use it in a safer way**, and that includes not carrying it on your person. Also know that when the cellphone is struggling to find reception or dialing, it produces more radiation. Some cellphones emit less radiation than others, and it is possible to buy low-EMF phones.

- **Minimize time and distance to all electric appliances:** while it's impossible to hold your electric toothbrush three feet away, you can use your electric blanket to heat up the bed and then turn it off. Considering ditching the baby monitor, microwave, and induction stove.
- **Switch to LED light bulbs.** They are lower-EMF and more efficient than CFLs.
- **Plug your electrical appliances into a power cord** and turn everything off at night, including, and most especially, your Wi-Fi router. It will save you from "phantom" electrical costs and reduce your EMF exposure at night, which is when some doctors say you are most vulnerable to its negative effects.
- **Advocate** keeping Wi-Fi out of your children's school.
- **Consider hiring a qualified technician** to do an EMF survey or help with shielding. This can give a more "tangible" picture of the strength and distribution of the "invisible" EMFs in the environment and locate sources that might otherwise be missed. Visit the International Institute for Building-Biology & Ecology at www.hbelc.org to find a qualified technician near you.

8. ♥ **Green your lifestyle habits.** Many small lifestyle habits that can help improve your indoor air quality are effective and cost almost nothing.

- **Properly dispose of all toxic household items**, including old appliances, batteries, paints, and toxic cleaning supplies, at an appropriate household hazardous waste facility. Often your local hardware store will take small appliances and light bulbs. Some provinces are beginning to enact extended producer responsibility programs that require companies to take back and recycle old products, so they (instead of you) are saddled with figuring out what to do with that old baby monitor, car seat, or plastic packaging. B.C., for example, has begun to do this with all electronics and packaging.
- **Do *not* smoke inside your home** and don't let others do it either. Even secondhand smoke on clothing can cause harm to a developing fetus. If you or another caregiver smokes, do it outside the home and change clothes frequently. If secondhand smoke is entering your home, consider investing in a high-quality HEPA air filter, which has minimal negative effects and can trap smoke, pollen, and dust. Beware, though, that even the best air filters won't fully clean the air. Also, many air filters create ozone, which at ground level is an irritant that can react with other household air pollutants to create toxins.
- **Dump the air freshener and odour eliminators.** Many air fresheners contain chemicals known to cause allergies and affect hormones and

reproductive development, particularly in babies and mamas-to-be. The only way to really clean the air is by introducing fresh air, so open the window. It can also help to use small bowls or packages of baking soda in the closet with the hockey gear or to sprinkle it on the carpets and vacuum it up. Essential oils are a wonderful way to introduce good smells that can also elevate mood. A diffuser is the most effective way to introduce bits of essential oils to the house, but you can also put some water and a few drops of essential oils in a spray bottle and spritz as wanted, add a few drops to your bowls of baking soda, or put some in water and heat it on your stove top.

- **Get a carbon monoxide detector** if you have an attached garage, gas or oil-fired furnace, or fireplace. Consider a **radon test**, especially if you have sunken rooms or a basement; a short-term radon detector kit is just $10 to $20.
- **Wet wipe your floors and surfaces** whenever possible to help remove dust and the corresponding toxins.
- **Get a few house plants**, as they can improve indoor air quality. Some of the best include aloe vera, bamboo palm, spider plants, chrysanthemums, red-edged or Warneckei dracaena, and weeping figs. There are houseplants that can be poisonous to children or pets if consumed, so buy safer options or ensure the plants are out of reach. Plant them in terracotta instead of plastic to prevent mould growth in the soil.
- **Open your windows whenever possible.** The outdoor air will greatly improve your indoor air quality. This is especially useful when running the dishwasher (which vaporizes the chemicals in the detergent and the water), while vacuuming, and when cooking.
- **Remove your shoes at the door.** They can track heavy metals, bacteria, and other pollutants into your home.

The Green Baby Shower Handbook

• •

There are few times as celebratory as the birth of a baby. It is the beginning of a new life and a new family configuration. Indeed, overnight, everything is about to be entirely different. It's a time to celebrate. It is also time to practise being the kind of parent you want to be. Throwing a baby shower that reflects your new family's values and interests is a great way to start.

Baby showers are, no surprise, a relatively new tradition brought to us via post–Second World War America. The culture of stuff, especially of stuff for children, was born at that time, and it wasn't born into a vacuum. Throughout time and across cultures, births have been celebrated. What most of these traditions have in common — which often gets omitted from today's baby shower — is the "mothering the mother" aspect. Nurtured mamas nurture healthy babies. This nurturing (both physical and psychological) is crucial in a mother's breastfeeding success, in helping prevent postpartum depression, and in how thoroughly she heals. In many cultures, in many times, this nurturing was particularly focused on the six weeks after giving birth. Women were encouraged to rest, to eat nutrient-rich foods, and to avoid stimulation. In these cultures, the celebrations often focused on helping the expectant mother prepare psychologically either for birth or for this postpartum period.

One of my friends who grew up in India had a baby shower to which everyone brought delicious homemade Indian treats for the expectant parents and bangles for the mother-to-be. These bangles were meant to be taken off, one by one, during the long hours of the birth. Another friend who had lived in the Middle East for many years chose to have a belly dancer at her baby shower. The women in attendance practised their "birthing" moves and then soaked the expectant mother's feet and massaged her hands. In some Afghani families and in some Jewish households, the celebration of birth happens after the baby arrives, and it usually involves bringing food for the entire family. The gifting of food is common among many of these traditions, and today many women continue this practice by asking guests to bring a frozen meal to their baby shower in preparation for the weeks to come.

A number of today's expectant moms are turning to something called a Blessing Way, which is supposedly derived from a Navajo tradition. It focuses on nurturing the woman in preparation for the birth, providing support from her community, and using some small "blessing" rituals. For instance, the women attending might share a few words of strength and encouragement

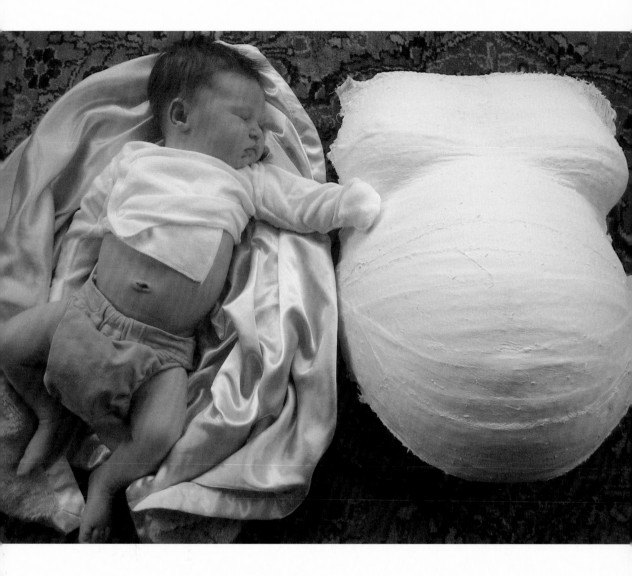

for the mom-to-be and then tie their wrists together with a beautiful "cord." Each woman will wear a bit of the cord as a bracelet, and when they are told that the expectant mother is in labour, they each cut their bracelet. The mom can wear the bracelet as a reminder of all those women cheering her on during this time. Or, something similar can be done with beeswax candles, which the woman burns during her labour and her friends and family burn in her honour as a way to share connection. Some women today use their blessing way to make a plaster cast of their pregnant belly, which can be a fun keepsake. Others simply ask their friends to bring a particularly meaningful note, prayer, or poem to share. These can be compiled into a beautiful book.

At my baby shower I incorporated a women-only part in which we painted my belly and shared positive birth experiences, and then had a larger celebration that included my husband and our many long-distance friends and family. We had everyone decorate small, triangular flags for the baby, and I strung them together to make a garland that still hangs in her room. For gifts, I asked people to bring one hand-me-down (a book or item) that had been really helpful or beloved in their own parenting or green life.

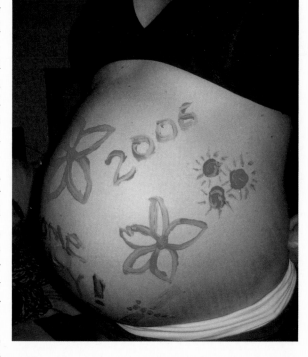

Whatever you choose to do, have a baby shower or blessing way or other celebration of some sort. Just because you're green, conscious, or into simpler living doesn't mean you shouldn't have fun and be supported. If we don't celebrate the big things, then how will we learn to honour the little things — the first step, the first tooth, the first time everybody sleeps through the night? Let the baby shower truly be a celebration of your intentions for parenting. Make it every bit as fun, green, and thoughtful as you want it to be. It'll be good practice for everything that comes after!

Getting support in the form of gifts of food, services, or a few truly needed items will let your community participate in supporting you during this time, without bogging you down with a bunch of stuff you don't really want or need. If you talk to experienced parents, they always have a list of the stuff they were tricked into buying or were given as a gift that they really didn't need. These things aren't just unnecessary and hard on the planet; they come to be annoying when you trip over them on the way to the bathroom in the middle of the night. There are also a few items that experienced parents will say they loved and never want to be without. Remember, having a baby is an exciting time, and people will want to give gifts to you. You just want to be very careful to direct your loving, well-intentioned family and friends away from the plastic baby-wipe warmer and toward that thing you really need. For ideas, see **What You Don't Need** and **Things New Parents Really Do Need** on the following pages.

The best way to get what you need is to ask for it. Registries can be a great help. Don't register at places like Babies "R" Us unless you are prepared for all the other stuff Great Aunt Matilda is going to grab for little Johnny when she goes there to get the one organic toy you wanted. Instead, register at your cool, local, green baby store. This way you can go there, see for yourself what you love, take a cloth diapering class, and then register for what you want online so that local friends can go to the store and out-of-town friends can just go online. Also, if something goes wrong and you want to return something, you already know you like lots of other items in the store.

If you want to compile a registry of a variety of specific green things, including a cloth diaper service, an organic mattress, and maybe even a homemade baby bed from Etsy, you can do this at www.babylist.com or at the nonprofit www.sokindregistry.org, where you can register for a donation (say, to a cause like supporting midwives in remote locations), for that organic mattress you've been wanting (but want a number of people to pitch in to help buy), or for time (getting someone to come Tuesday to do laundry, Wednesday to make dinner, and Thursday to hold the baby so you can take a shower). Canada also has a number of websites full of great green items, such as www.lifewithoutplastic.com, www.matraea.com, and www.well.ca. Even better, find a little green boutique near you that also has an online registry or website so that you can exchange in person those things you inevitably get but don't want.

What You Don't Need

Big and plastic, ugly and impossible to dispose of properly, or just designed to be useless after a year, these are among the many things you don't need to receive at a baby shower:

1. The Diaper Genie. This is a plastic garbage can just for diapers. By some unknown magic, it twists the diapers into tight little sausages that are supposed to stink less, but it requires lots of plastic and specially designed bags to do it. As if you need another thing to run out to buy at midnight.
2. A plastic wash tub. That's what sinks are for.
3. A changing table. They are one of the top polluters in a home, and six months later they serve no purpose.
4. A baby wipe warmer. They spread the chemicals from baby wipes all around the house.
5. Polyester baby pajamas. They are oh so cute, but they often contain chemical flame retardants.
6. Plastic toys.

7. Also, wait and see before you buy strollers, baby monitors, and baby clothes. What you think you want and what you end up using can be very different. I know that the impulse to buy that beautiful, expensive (it's got a matching cup holder!) baby stroller is nearly overwhelming. However, for the first few months you will likely just use the stroller that your car seat clicks into or you will keep your baby close in the sling. Then, you may just find you don't need to buy a stroller at all because someone gave you a simple umbrella stroller and you love it.

Things New Parents Really Do Need

You will be given lots and lots of things, including a million baby clothes, so ask for those things that you aren't likely to be given and are really sure you want. There are a few things that will make life so much easier, and you will love having them in your life.

1. Services such as a postpartum doula, food delivery, or just someone to wash the clothes and fold the laundry (no one has ever regretted a little extra help).
2. A really natural place for baby to sleep: a crib with a natural mattress, an all-wood co-sleeper or bassinet with the same kind of mattress but smaller, or just an organic wool puddle pad to put under the baby as she sleeps in your bed.
3. Cloth diapers. I suggest paying for a service for the first three months, when you will be changing the baby all the time. The service washes the diapers for you and takes them back when you are ready for bigger or different diapers. There are dozens of sites in Canada where you can register for cloth diapers and for "trial packs," where you try different types of cloth diapers before you commit to one. Every major city has a store selling cloth diapers, and online stores include (among many) www.bumbini.ca, www.calgaryclothdiaperdepot.com, www.ottawaclothdiapers.com, www.theclothdiapersource.ca, www.jilliansdrawers.com, www.newandgreen.com, and www.littlemonkeystore.com.
4. Baby slings and carriers. A basic sling and a soft-sided carrier such as an Ergo- or Mei Tai–style are extremely useful tools for the modern parent.
5. Sleep sack or swaddle. There are all-cotton, organic swaddles with Velcro. They are the best thing ever for swaddling, and swaddling is the best thing ever to get your new baby to sleep.
6. Healthy and organic teas, salves, and sitz bath ingredients to help you to heal and your baby to get the most natural start.

7. Baby socks. Seriously, at least six million pairs, in a variety of sizes, but ones that *actually stay on*.

8. A few good books. I highly recommend *Green Mama: Giving Your Child a Healthy Start and a Greener Future* (shameless self-promotion!). Or, see the end of this book for more great books on topics such as nutrition, vaccinations, sleep, parenting, and more. And visit me online at www.thegreenmama.com for more book recommendations and resources.

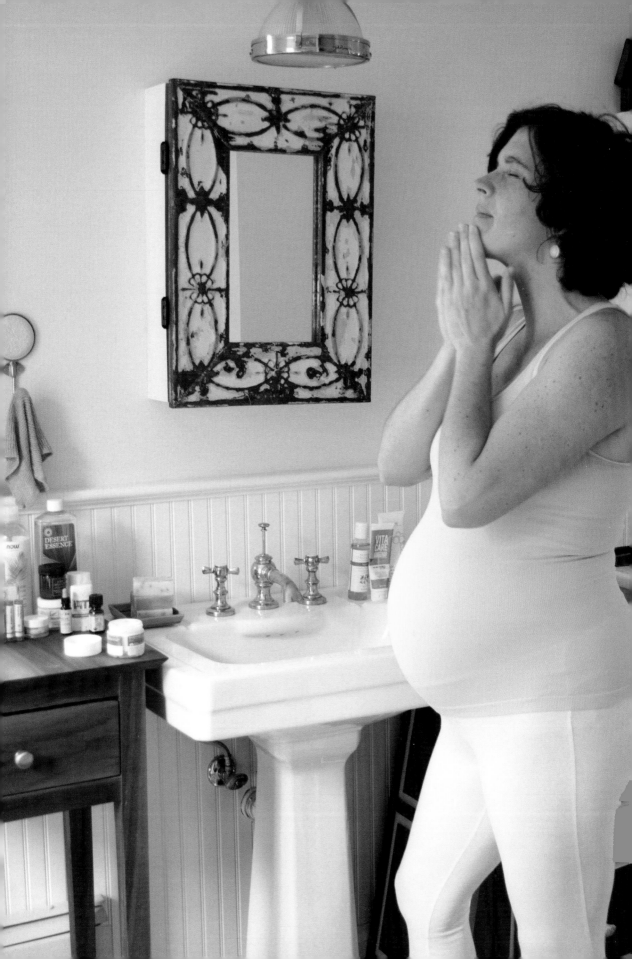

chapter five

Greening Your Beauty Care

· ·

I celebrated my first pregnancy with a trip to the nail salon and I dyed my hair during my second. And that's me: the woman who researches toxin-free living. We all have blind spots. I doubt I am the only woman for whom some of them are particularly stark around beauty care. I have long since cleaned up my act as far as deodorants, makeup, and shampoo are concerned, but there were some things that just took a little longer.

When I was writing my first book, one of my most respected environmental heroes read the book to provide a blurb (read on to see who!). His one bit of advice was that I needed to warn women about just how dangerous hair dyes are. I took his research and comments to heart. I have never dyed my hair since, even with supposedly natural dyes. I figured if I couldn't learn to love my hair as it was then, what would happen when I went grey? I have since spoken with a lot of my most health-oriented peers — including some interviewed in this book — and it turns out that hair dying is a challenge for even some of the healthiest women — even, and often especially, during pregnancy. "I couldn't bear to be pregnant and have grey hair," said one, and, "I didn't want to look like I was the grandma holding the baby," said another.

What are your blind spots? Is it that antiperspirant, the signature perfume, or that perfect lipstick? For most things there are greener alternatives. But it takes time to get used to seeing ourselves without hair colour from the bottle. Or for others to get used to the fact that, while you can definitely still smell good without antiperspirant, you may never be able to wear that polyester blouse during a presentation (man-made fibres mixed with stress equals armpit sweat, no matter how much natural deodorant you use!). Or, as another friend advised me, you are just in the habit of seeing yourself with eyeliner and mascara.

For me, at first, I simply changed to greener options, but eventually I plan on getting used to seeing my face "naked." Luckily, I've been assured that this year the fashion "in" is the natural, no-makeup look. In the meantime, there are many healthier and extremely effective options as close as your local drugstore or favourite natural grocery. If there was ever a time to battle the beast of the beauty care industry, at least in your own personal choices, it's during pregnancy.

The Research

Here it is in plain language: we put many of the worst-known toxins on our skin and in our hair. The average woman applies more than 500 chemicals every day. Our skin is porous and vulnerable, so 60 to 90 percent of what goes on it can end up entering our bloodstream. This is particularly a problem during pregnancy and breastfeeding, when what enters your bloodstream can pass through the placental barrier and into your baby, where neither the blood-brain barrier nor the organs of detoxification are fully formed. It takes very, very little exposure to affect a forming child for a lifetime.

It isn't just our guts that have coevolved with bacteria and other microbes. Our skin, too, is a microcosm of about a trillion microbes — including bacteria, parasites, fungi, and even animal species — that have co-evolved along with us. And there is a great deal of difference between the microbes found in our armpits versus those found on our faces. The variance is due to the amount of light, hair, or oil that a part of the body has or receives. The microbes don't just sit on top, either, but penetrate down through the layers to the subcutaneous fat. They also change during a person's life: a hormonal teenager's microbes will look very different from a postmenopausal woman's. As with the gut microbiome research, we still don't know what an "ideal" skin microbiome is, but, also similar to the gut microbiome, a healthy skin microbiome is an effective defensive layer against pathogens. Some of the skin microbes are better defenders than others, some are smellier than others, and some are better communicators — sending messages to the immune system to dampen or increase inflammation. As with the gut, it is assumed that a rich diversity of microbes is probably better.

We are beginning to understand through studies that our cosmetic products are capable of affecting this microbiome, sometimes quite dramatically, as in the case of routine users of antiperspirants and deodorants, who showed significant differences in types and quantity of bacteria present based on product use. Interestingly, among other findings, antiperspirant wearers were found to have significantly more opportunistic bacteria than either deodorant or no-underarm-cosmetic wearers.

An imbalanced microbiome, or skin dysbiosis, may be associated with diseases of the skin that include acne, allergies, dandruff, eczema, psoriasis, and yeast and fungal infections. Antibacterial soaps, topical steroids, and even internal antibiotics can damage the skin microbiome. Exposure to antimicrobial household products has been shown to lead to allergy symptoms like wheezing, runny nose, and congestion in children.

Cosmetic Penetration

What we put in our skin and on our hair ends up in our bloodstream, and from there it can enter our growing baby-to-be. Cosmetic ingredients are designed to do just that: penetrate. These ingredients are routinely found in human bodies, including those of newborn babies. Phthalates and triclosan are found in the urine of almost everyone, parabens and talc have been found in breast tumour tissue, and persistent fragrance components like musk xylene have been discovered in human fat tissue. Smaller is not always better: nanoparticles and micro-beads are proving to be able to penetrate right through both the blood-brain barrier in an adult and through the placenta.

Just a little bigger than nanoparticles are the tiny plastic micro-beads that are found in body scrubs, bath products, facial cleansers, creams, deodorant, fluoridated toothpaste, and even products sold specifically for babies and pregnant women. Micro-beads are just the most recent icon of a growing global plastic problem, the products that have increased more than sixfold since 1975, and which is estimated at around 288 million metric tonnes a year. The problem with plastic is that, while it can photodegrade (get smaller and smaller), it can't biodegrade. No natural process can break plastic down into simpler compounds, even if it starts microscopically small. In the environment, micro plastics can react with and absorb other environmental pollutants, break down and release their own plasticizer components, or settle into sediment. They have been found all over the globe in deep sea sediments, ice cores, on the beaches of the Great Lakes, and in supposedly pristine fresh and seawater sources in the most remote regions of Canada. They are found in zooplankton, mussels, and fish. They can move across the food web between species that eat each other. They move from the GI tract to other tissues and cells. Perhaps most troubling, they can absorb other pollutants — such as chemical flame retardants, pesticides, and triclosan — and then release them into their new animal host, where they are able to effect embryonic development. There is good news. Canada and the U.S. are banning micro-beads from most toiletries starting in July 2018 and from nonprescription drugs and toothpaste in July 2019.

Dying for a Better Hair Colour

"I believe [hair dye] is more pernicious than women (and men) understand, know, or are told," says environmentalist and author Paul Hawken. "Coal tar dye molecules are so small they pass transdermally into the bloodstream. From that point, there is no knowing what happens in terms of their impact. With hair dye we are doing to our heads what we are doing to our earth. Pouring chemicals on it in order to get it to be the way we want it to be."

It is clearly an environmental issue: 90 percent of hair dye ends up going down the drain into aquatic environments. Yet, again, what is an environmental issue ends up as a human issue. "This is a ticking time bomb in women's health," says Hawken.

Hair dyes being advertised as natural and organic, even by recognizable companies such as Aveda and Madison Reed, are still using the same main ingredients. "All they are doing is pulling ammonia or parabens out, adding some essential oils or ginseng, but not changing the main ingredients because they cannot." The main ingredients of concern in permanent hair colour are paraphenylenediamine (PPD) — which is made from 4-nitrochlorobenzene — and 2,5-diaminotoluene (PTD), the same chemicals used to make cartridge toner, car tires, polyurethane, colour film developer, and more.

"In research I have done with women, many know in some way that hair dyeing is bad. They almost do not want to know more because then they would have to stop using it. These are women (and moms) who use only pure water, organic food, et cetera, who are impeccable in their daily life but they cannot let their hair go grey because they are professionals or in companies where it would disadvantage them."

Greener Beauty Care to the Rescue

When it comes to cosmetics, consumers are getting smart. Greener cosmetics are becoming increasingly popular. The global demand for greener personal care products is expected to reach US$13.2 billion by 2018, in a beauty market that is already worth $170 billion annually. There are a number of retailers helping make the consumer's job easier. Whole Foods has been leading the charge on removing the worst cosmetics from its shelves, and Loblaws, one of Canada's largest retailers, announced it is phasing out phthalates, triclosan, and micro-beads from its store brands.

Wherever there is a lot of money, there are also less-than-scrupulous companies hoping to get some of the reward without doing all of the work. Thus, it's still important to look for trustworthy green labels and avoid companies that are greenwashing (see sidebar).

USDA Organic and Other Trustworthy Skincare Labels

The gold standard of green cosmetic labels is the **USDA Organic** label. In order for a product to get the USDA organic seal, the product must contain at least 95 percent organic food-grade ingredients — yup, that's right; it must be organic and edible to get this label. The other 5 percent of non-organic ingredients is restricted to food-safe standards, too. That means there are some things that will just never be able to be certified as USDA Organic because, while as safe as they can be, they aren't edible: things like mascara, sunblock, and nail polish.

There are some second-tier standards that allow a number of synthetics and more processing — and, thus, more impurities — but that still keep you safer from most of the worst offenders and the sheer volume of chemicals that can appear in regular cosmetics. These labels include the NSF label and the NPA labels. The new COSMetic Organic Standard (COSMOS) in Europe brought together

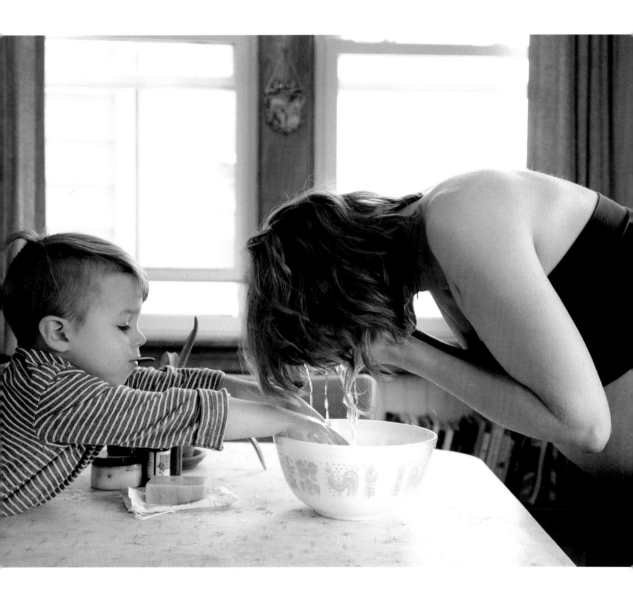

a number of Europe's green labels under one harmonized label. This standard allows a maximum of 5 percent synthetic content, and a minimum of 20 percent by volume must be organic. They also offer a more lenient "natural" standard. All COSMOS-labelled cosmetics must adhere to the precautionary principle, and the product cannot contain any nano-materials or GMOs or have undergone irradiation or animal testing. Other international labels include the Soil Association in the UK, BDIH in Germany, and ACO and NASAA in Australia. These labels, however, allow some synthetic preservatives and petrochemical ingredients. Standards to avoid because they aren't stringent enough to be meaningful include Oasis, EcoCert, and Natrue (other than their highest three-star rating).

greening your beauty care 133

How to Green Your Beauty Care

Here are a series of action steps listed from ♥♥♥ (biggest impact, and possibly more work) to ♥ (quick and easy) to help make your beauty care routine as healthy as possible for you and your future children.

1. ♥♥♥ **Read the label.** The USDA Organic label is the safest, highest standard for beauty care items, but there are other guidelines available for beauty care items not likely to be edible. When you are shopping outside the USDA Organic label, take the list of 20 ingredients to always avoid (see the **Green Mama-to-Be*ware* appendix) and ensure the item is free of those ingredients. Beware, though! In the United States, beauty care products don't need to reveal their ingredients on the label, and in Canada items like toothpaste, sunscreen, anti-aging moisturizer, antiperspirant, and anything else with a therapeutic purpose doesn't need to reveal its ingredients either.

2. ♥♥ **Rethink your big users.** If you like to use perfume regularly or apply skin cream as soon as you exit the shower, then apply your new label-reading talents to these favourites and hold your biggest users to the highest standards (at least for all of the pregnancy). Remember, however, that it may not be that easy to get to the bottom of what's in your cosmetic products even in Canada, because of "hidden" ingredients. There are websites, like the Environmental Working Group's Skin Deep database (www.ewg.org/skindeep), that have done the work of revealing and rating thousands of cosmetic and consumer products.

3. ♥♥ **Filter your shower water.** Chlorine — and some other toxins found in water — are readily absorbed via the lungs and skin. It's estimated that half of the average person's exposure to chlorine comes through the skin. It is known that chlorine can have an antibacterial effect and disrupt the microbiome. Chloroform gas, a known carcinogen that is related to airborne chlorine, is found in just about every North American home, presumably originating from tap water. When chlorine enters the body through the lungs and skin, it enters into the bloodstream. Chlorine can also be an issue in swimming pools; it is possible to find non-chlorinated pools and freshwater swimming holes, and even just an outdoor pool will reduce exposure. A simple shower filter will remove most of the chlorine, and most heavy metals, in your shower. They install easily (even I can do it) just above your shower head and cost around $20. A similar "ball" version is available for your bathtub as well.

Greenwashing

Greenwashing is when a company or products pretends it's healthier, more ecological, and socially conscious than it really is. According to *The Sins of Greenwashing*, more than 95 percent of companies are committing at least one of the greenwashing sins. This often happens in industries where labelling regulations are weak or confusing, which is certainly the case in the beauty industry. Beware of non-regulated but green-sounding language like "Natural," "With Real Natural Ingredients," "Dermatologist Tested," "Herbal," and even "Organic" if it isn't backed up by the USDA organic label. Also beware of companies touting irrelevant health claims such as "Supports Green Energy," "Profits go to Breast Cancer Research," or "Recyclable Packaging." Instead, look for trust-worthy labels such as the USDA Organic label. (Unfortunately, the Canadian organic/biologique label is not currently applied to any body care products at all.)

4. ♥♥ **Skip the hair dye or go for a greener option.** It's not enough for a label to say "natural" or "organic" on hair dye (unless certified by a third-party such as the USDA or COSMOS). Greener options are often called stains or washes, and they coat the hair shaft rather than being absorbed into it. That means that they aren't permanent and, unfortunately, aren't that effective at covering grey. Ingredients might include henna, vegetable-based colours, and hydrogen peroxide. But beware that hair dyes don't need to disclose all of their ingredients, and even henna can contain paraphenylenediamine (a particular problem when seeking darker colours). You can make your own hair tint at home using walnut shells, turmeric, or beet juice.

5. ♥♥ **Forgo antibacterial products.** Soaps, deodorants, and hand sanitizers are just as good at cleaning, but without the same repercussions to the microbiome. Triclosan, the main ingredient in antibacterial hand soaps and other antibacterial products, is a pesticide, and its use has been linked to the development of antibacterial-resistant superbugs.

6. ♥♥ **Find better toothpaste.** It's not just about fluoride. Toothpaste can contain SLS, triclosan, aluminum, and other yucky ingredients. Greener,

The Not-So-Hot List

In Canada, the Chemical Management Plan does not oversee cosmetic chemicals. Instead, that responsibility belongs to Health Canada as part of the Food and Drug Act and the Cosmetic Regulations. Health Canada has developed the Cosmetic Ingredient Hotlist as the first step in the process of protecting citizens from the worst of these chemicals. The Hotlist has limitations.

The list has no legal authority and cannot be enforced. For instance, coal tar or p-phenylenediamine — used in making hair dyes and some shampoos and lotions — is a known human carcinogen linked to tumours and cancer in the lungs, kidneys, and bladder. It is on the Hotlist. Yet it's allowed to be used with a safety stamp warning on the package that warns about skin and eye irritation. The warning doesn't even mention the known carcinogenic aspects. Not to mention that if you are getting your hair dyed in the salon, you may never read the warning label anyway. There are no other limits, such as on how much of the toxic chemicals can be used, or limits on what other toxins they can be used with, or warnings about use during pregnancy. It's all left up to the manufacturer and whether they want to expose consumers to that Hotlist item or voluntarily remove it from their formula. While the Hotlist points to about 500 chemicals that we consider too dangerous for routine exposure, the list doesn't keep us safe.

Even suspected toxins aren't put on the list until after the research has been done, and it's slow. Of the 4,000 chemicals that are thought to potentially be eligible for the list, only a fraction have been tested. The vast majority of chemicals used in cosmetics have not yet been tested.

The list isn't set up to include toxic impurities or by-products. For instance, while formaldehyde is on the list, the formaldehyde-releasing preservative DMDM hydantoin is not.

Canada is moving in the right direction, albeit slowly, with the 2006 requirement to label cosmetic ingredients. These aren't the same as warning labels, but it does mean that many cosmetic ingredients can be found in the fine print and, if you know what you are looking for, avoided. Unfortunately, those unintentional ingredients such as formaldehyde won't appear on the ingredient label, nor will the "trade secret" chemical components of fragrances or parfums, nor will the ingredients in products deemed "therapeutic," including antiperspirants, toothpaste, hand sanitizers, anti-aging lotions, and just about anything with sunscreen.

more natural options are getting easier to find and are available at most retailers in Canada. Many voluntarily reveal their ingredients, point out that they are free of all the worst no-no's, and may even be certified organic. Two greener, Canadian-made options I recommend are Green Beaver and Druide. Or you can even make your own toothpaste.

While upgrading your toothpaste, also look at your dental floss. Most dental floss is made from petroleum-based nylon and is coated in both petroleum-based wax and PTFE, the toxic material used in nonstick pans. There are uncoated options, as well as dental floss made with natural materials like silk.

7. ♥♥ **Forget antiperspirants and find a healthy deodorant alternative.** Antiperspirants work by blocking the sweat glands, and deodorants work by trying to prevent or kill the bacteria that cause odour. Sweating is one of the ways our body detoxifies. Adding a known neurotoxin day after day to the vulnerable skin around our armpits, while decreasing a known toxin exit route, isn't a great idea. Especially while pregnant. We know that aluminum is able to penetrate through the skin in small amounts and enter the bloodstream and from there pass through the placental barrier. There are no safe levels for a fetus. As well, antiperspirant manufacturers aren't required to list ingredients, and products can contain many of the **Twenty Concerning Cosmetic Ingredients** (see the **Green Mama-to-Be**ware appendix). There are safer deodorants that use baking soda or cornstarch, essential oils, vinegar, and naturally antibacterial oils to work, and many of these are made in Canada. It's even possible to make your own.

8. ♥ **Use greener makeup.** There are a growing number of cosmetics being made using mineral- and food-based pigments and without the addition of petrochemicals, fragrance, or the worst of the synthetic preservatives. A number of these companies are based in Canada. You can shop for greener makeup online or at your favourite health food store or natural apothecary, like the Canadian-based Finlandia.

The DIY Green Beauty Care Handbook

· ·

Do-it-yourself (DIY) is an economical and fun way to reduce your exposure to the worst chemicals in beauty care products. When you do it yourself, you know exactly what is going into a product and you can spend all the money on getting the best ingredients and none supporting the multi-million-dollar advertising budgets of big beauty care companies. You can't go too wrong with good ingredients, whether you are a bit more maverick like me, just throwing any old stuff in a jar and calling it skin oil, or a real DIY apothecary, like those who helped with the recipes and recommendations in this handbook. (Thank you, Summer Knight of Native Formula [nativeformula.com] and Jingo and Piper of Neitra Body Botanicals [www.neitra.ca].)

Best Oils for Skincare

Remember, as with all fats, it is particularly important to buy the highest quality organic and unrefined oils possible.

- **Avocado oil:** Rich in vitamins (including E) and essential fatty acids (EFA). Absorbed easily, and slows the progress of wrinkles. Regenerative.
- **Apricot oil:** Softens skin. Good for scalp. Easily absorbed.
- **Sweet almond oil:** Absorbs well, soothing, and rich in vitamins A and B and EFAs. Good for many skin types. Very little odour.
- **Calendula oil (a blend):** Healing and anti-inflammatory. Great for cracked and damaged skin, rashes, wounds, scars, and eczema.
- **Cocoa butter:** High in antioxidants and fatty acids. Builds elasticity.
- **Coconut oil:** Emollient. High in saturated fats, EFAs, and vitamin E, with antibacterial, antimicrobial, and antifungal properties. Mild sunscreen properties. Helps with rashes and acne, but slightly comedogenic.
- **Grape seed oil:** Light and thin and high in EFAs.
- **Jojoba oil:** Good for oily and dehydrated skin, acne, dryness, inflammation, eczema, psoriasis, and achy muscles. Balancing and anti-inflammatory. Rich in vitamins and minerals.
- **Olive oil:** Moisturizing. Can be used directly on hair, lips, and skin.
- **Rosehip oil:** A "dry" penetrating oil, high in EFAs and antioxidants. Good for sun damage, scars, and wrinkles. Stimulates collagen.

- **Sesame oil:** Anti-inflammatory and antioxidant. Helps with skin regeneration and removing toxins. Mild sunscreen properties.
- **Shea butter:** Excellent emollient properties.
- **St. John's wort oil (a blend):** Can help with nerve pain, shingles, wounds, and tissue trauma.
- **Sunflower oil:** Light, with many vitamins. Good for massage.

Body Care Recipes and Tips

Makeup Remover

This one is so simple. Use a vegetable or fruit oil of your choice on a cloth or cotton ball to help dissolve mascara or other makeup.

Hair Mask

Hair is best nurtured the same way the rest of us is: through good nutrition. Food, however, can also be used on the hair to add a bit of extra lustre. Apply avocado mixed with honey and a few drops of lavender for 20 minutes and

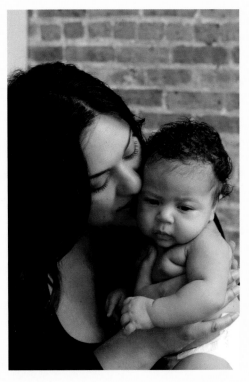

then rinse off. Or try this recipe: mix equal parts jojoba oil, avocado oil, and coconut oil (coconut oil can be warmed by placing it in a metal bowl over hot water). Pour the mixture into a container of choice. Thoroughly saturate the entire strand of hair when applying, and leave for at least 20 minutes. For greater penetration, put a shower cap on and sit in the sun, use a hair dryer, or leave it on overnight. Wash and rinse as normal.

Easy Body Butter (created by Neitra Body Botanicals)

Use equal parts of coconut oil, shea butter, and cocoa butter. Melt these three ingredients (use a metal bowl over warm water and stir constantly); once melted and blended together, remove from heat. If you want, you can add a few drops of your favourite pregnancy-safe essential oil at this point. Pour into a container and leave to set before using.

Lip Balm

Ingredients:
2 teaspoons (10g) pure cosmetic-grade beeswax
2 tablespoons (30ml) sweet almond oil or coconut oil
Optional: 2 drops vitamin E oil (you can get this by puncturing a vitamin capsule), 5 drops essential oil (orange, lemon, and peppermint are nice choices), or 1/4 teaspoon grated natural mineral lipstick for colour.

Directions:
1. Slowly warm the beeswax in a double boiler just until it melts, then add in the oils. (If you want to add colour, add the lipstick while the mixture is still warm.) Mix well.
2. Set aside until lukewarm; add optional essential oils and vitamin E. Pour into a small container and let sit before using.

Essential Oils: Which One Is Right for You?

All Skin Types
True lavender (flowering tops): antimicrobial, antiseptic, healing to skin; aids in cell regeneration
Carrot oil (dried fruit seeds): antiseptic, tonic; can be used for revitalizing and toning
Lemon (outer part of peel): antimicrobial, antiseptic, astringent

For Dry Skin
Sandalwood (roots and heartwood): astringent, bactericidal, tonic, strengthening; good for moisturizing dry, cracked, or chapped skin

For Normal Skin
Geranium (leaves, stalks, flowers): astringent, anti-inflammatory, tonic, wound healing

For Oily Skin
Bergamot (from the peel): antiseptic, tonic, wound healing

For Sensitive Skin
Roman chamomile (flowers): healing, anti-inflammatory, antiseptic

For Mature Skin
Frankincense (gum resin): anti-inflammatory, antiseptic, tonic; good for blemishes, dry skin, and wrinkles
Orange blossom (flowers): antiseptic, bactericidal, tonic; good for complexion

Cleansing Facial Oil and Moisturizer (created by Neitra Body Botanicals)

Blend 3 parts rose hip oil with 1 part jojoba oil. Add a few drops of your favourite essential oil to the blend.

Magnesium Oil

Your body needs magnesium, and it is particularly well absorbed through the skin (as magnesium chloride). Healthy magnesium levels can help with arthritic pain, muscle and joint pain, depression, insomnia, stress, and balancing blood sugar levels. It can even help with ADHD and learning disorders. Beware, though, because the first few times you use it, it stings! **(For children, dilute with water by half.)** Spray magnesium on your body daily (I recommend spraying on the bottom of your feet and armpits as it is readily absorbed in both places). Start with six squirts and build up to more.

Ingredients:
1/2 cup magnesium chloride flakes (these can be found in most drug stores as well as online from sources such as Ancient Minerals)
1/2 cup (125ml) purified or distilled water

Directions:
1. Boil the water.
2. Add magnesium chloride flakes and stir well until dissolved.
3. When cool, transfer to a glass spray bottle.

Deodorant Tips and Recipes

Making your own deodorant can be as simple as mixing 1/8 teaspoon of baking soda with a few drops of water (moisten, don't dissolve). Add a pinch of cornstarch and a drop of essential oil to the mix, and you have an odour-fighting, nice smelling, easy concoction. Increase the basic recipe and store it in a jar. The final result is softer than typical deodorant, but applies easily with fingers or cloth to the underarms.

To make a final product that's more solid (at least in cooler climates), blend 6 tablespoons coconut oil with 2 tablespoons baking soda. Add 10 to 15 drops of your favourite essential oils (e.g., tea tree oil, lavender, or wild orange). If you find baking soda irritating, try the same recipe using arrowroot instead of baking soda.

Or take your magnesium oil (which can also help prevent body odour), add essential oils (10 drops of essential oil for 2 ounces of magnesium oil), and spray on!

Springtime Cleansing Facial and Body Toning Mist (created by Native Formula)

Ingredients:
1/4 cup (60ml) hibiscus tea from organic dried herbs, or prepackaged organic tea (Hibiscus has softening, firming, and lifting qualities. You can use chamomile instead if you have any skin irritations or you want a calming effect.)
1/4 cup (60ml) aloe vera juice
1/4 cup (60ml) witch hazel
1 tablespoon (15ml) organic apple cider vinegar

Personal Lubricants

Many women find that when they are pregnant they produce more natural lubrication along with all those other fluids they are busy producing. When trying to get pregnant or adding lubrication to your post-conception intercourse, it pays to be particularly aware of the toxins and irritants in most name-brand lubricants, including those especially designed to "enhance" fertility. Bacterial vaginosis can result from vaginal irritation and has been linked to lower rates of fertility and early miscarriage. Common lubricant ingredients to avoid include chlorhexidine, glycerin, parabens, petroleum by-products and silicone-based ingredients (including methyl polysiloxane and dimethicone), phenoxyethanol, and propylene glycol.

Instead of name-brand lubricants that may contain harmful or unnecessary ingredients, I recommend using natural oils such as canola (which Dr. Oz calls "sperm-friendly"), olive oil, and cocoa butter. For those using latex condoms, try plain yogourt or aloe vera gel.

Directions:
1. Brew your tea in purified or distilled water for 15–20 minutes.
2. Once cooled, combine the tea, aloe vera juice, witch hazel, and apple cider vinegar in a glass bottle with a spritzer top. Shake well.

Can be used all over. In warmer months, store in the fridge for a cool mist. Use within two weeks.

Easy Rose Toner (created by Neitra Body Botanicals)

Blend equal parts distilled water with rose distillate (rose water). Add a few drops of your favourite essential oil. Pour into a glass bottle with a spritzer top.

Fairy Kisses Facial Serum (created by Native Formula)

This is such an easy, light, and nourishing moisturizer. Try using while your skin is slightly damp from the toner above.

Ingredients:
1 tablespoon (15ml) avocado oil
1 tablespoon (15ml) apricot oil
2 tablespoons (30ml) aloe vera gel
3–5 drops of pure essential oil (optional)

Place all of the ingredients in a small glass bottle, shake, and enjoy! You may add essential oils of your choice, but opt not to if you have overly sensitive skin.

Mama Bear Belly Rub and Balm (created by Native Formula)

Ingredients:
1 teaspoon (5g) beeswax
1 tablespoon (15g) cocoa butter
1 1/2 teaspoon (7g) shea butter
7 tablespoons (105ml) oil (pick a favourite or a mix from the **Best Oils for Skincare** list)
1 teaspoon (5ml) raw manuka honey
1 vitamin E capsule, or a few drops of vitamin E oil
10–15 drops of pure essential oil of your choice

Directions:
1. Place the first four ingredients in a clean glass jar.
2. Take a medium saucepan and fill with about 5 centimetres of water. Bring to a simmer.
3. Once the water has reached a low simmer, set your jar in the middle of the pot of water. Let the butters and oils slowly warm.
4. Once the mixture has melted completely, remove the jar carefully using a towel and set on your countertop. Add the manuka honey, vitamin E, and essential oils. Swirl about to gently mix. Once mixed, quickly pour the melted balm into the tin or jar of your choice. If you notice separation developing, just pop the jar back into the hot water for a few more minutes to let it melt again. Take out, swirl, and pour into a container.

DIY Sunscreen

Ingredients:
1/2 cup (125ml) olive oil
1/4 cup (55g) coconut oil
1/4 cup (57g) beeswax
2 tablespoons (27g) shea butter

2 tablespoons (30g) zinc oxide (high quality)

Optional: 2–3 drops of an essential oil that is safe for use in the sun (not phototoxic), such as cold-pressed mandarin, sweet orange, or tangerine, or steam-distilled bergamot or lemon

Directions:

1. In a double boiler (or a jar in a pan of water over low heat), melt the oils, beeswax, and shea butter together.
2. Once melted, remove the mixture from the heat and let cool to room temperature. Whisk in the zinc oxide at this point, being very careful not to breathe in the fumes. You may also add the essential oil at this point, if using.
3. Store in a glass container in the fridge between uses. It is not waterproof, so reapply often.

Shortcut DIY Sunscreen Recipe

Take your favourite natural skin cream, baby's bum balm, or belly rub and whip in 2 tablespoons (30g) of zinc oxide.

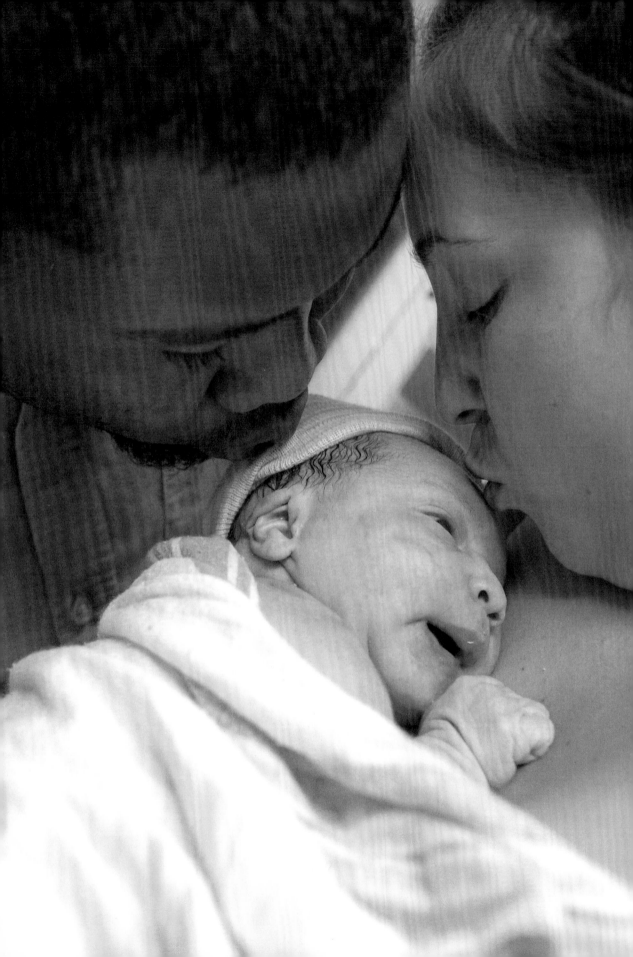

Greening Birth, Breastfeeding, and Beyond

• •

My first baby was born in Chicago, at home. When I would mention home birth in that city at the time, it was akin to saying, "I like to fly stunt planes. Wanna set yourself on fire and take a ride with me?" Mothers were aghast: I must be nuts, or at least horribly anti-establishment.

My second baby was born in Vancouver, British Columbia. There, home birth is just part of the culture. In my yoga class, three out of the four pregnant women were planning home births; the fourth was working with midwives in a hospital. Okay, so it was a yoga class; not exactly a random sampling, but still impressive.

Then I moved to Guatemala, where everybody was having home births because there wasn't any other option, which is a problem when things go awry and there are complications. In the little town where I lived, two women lost their lives in childbirth on the same night.

Today I live on a remote island with no hospital or midwife, and the women there must choose between going to the nearest town (two ferries away), to a facility with one of the highest Caesarean section rates in the country, or going it alone at home. That's not a choice I'd like to have to make, and it reinforces the fact that one of the challenges Canada faces is providing birth options across provinces and territories, including in its many remote communities.

Birth is both an end and a beginning. Or, as a midwife described it to me, "It's part biology and part magic." With birth, you are no longer the sole creator of your child's environment. I have seen many women become passionate about "Mother Earth" and healing her food, water, and air after they have given birth, as they realize that their child now inhabits a much larger womb that is increasingly precarious.

When I looked into my babies' eyes for the first time, I knew love in a new way. Elation, relief, and joy flooded through me, and I quickly forgot the discomfort of pregnancy and the pain of labour. It was all worth it for this moment of bliss and this child to love forever. That moment — and the hormones, brain changes, and other physiological processes of the birth — helped carry me through many of the hard moments of recovering from childbirth and managing modern-day parenting.

The Research

We are very fortunate to live at a time and in a place where women and babies are less likely to die in childbirth. Unfortunately, where a woman lives and her societal status still influences those statistics dramatically. The United States, with all of its medical advances, still has one of the highest maternal death rates in the developed world, and it's getting worse. Canada has half the rate of maternal death, with only seven out of every 100,000 women dying from birth-related causes. Unfortunately, our rate hasn't improved over the last 15 years, while countries like Austria, Czech Republic, Finland, Iceland, Italy, Kuwait, Poland, Sweden, and Greece have managed to get their rates down to four deaths or fewer per 100,000 — in many cases a reduction by more than half — over the same period. Infant mortality rates in Canada continue to be four times higher for some First Nations populations, further indicating that birth outcomes are influenced by more than just the country in which a person lives.

Even though much of the science of pregnancy and even birth is still unfolding, there are things we know that can make the time of birth and the days that come directly after it easier and healthier for both mother and baby. One of these is to have a natural birth, if possible. While birth, like breastfeeding, is the most natural thing in the world, today it takes preparation to have a truly physiological birth. In some hospitals in North America, the first-time mother is more likely to end up with a Caesarean section (C-section) than she is a vaginal birth, despite her desires. As the Matraea midwives say, "You wouldn't just sign up for a marathon the day before, never train, and show up and expect to do well." Similarly, getting a great birth takes a little preparation of your body, mind, and your partner or support, and it is very important to have a provider that, like a great coach, is willing to work with you to achieve the best possible birth for all involved.

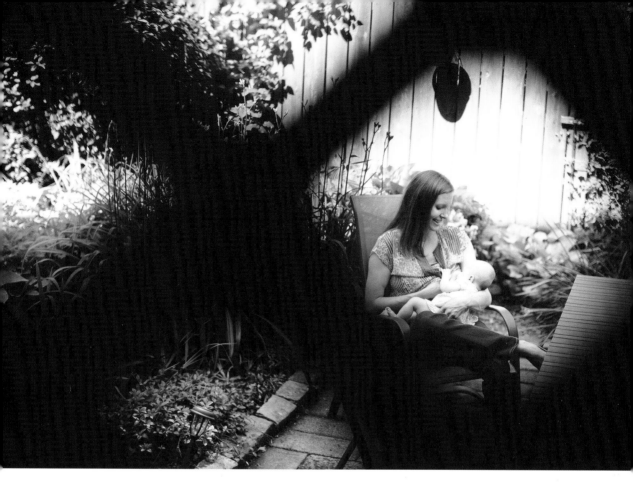

"All that counts is that the baby is healthy" is what many women are told and believe about birth. But the research reveals something quite different: *a woman's experience matters.* This is because a woman who is involved and empowered in her birth is more likely to have a vaginal birth. This increases the woman's chances of recovering speedily, of successfully breastfeeding, and of having subsequent healthy pregnancies and babies. Also, it decreases the chances of a woman suffering the negative effects possible with a C-section, including longer and more painful recoveries, and other serious health problems. The more we learn about the microbiome and the role of the birth canal, the more we see that birth itself is perfectly designed to enhance a number of other processes that set the child up for future health.

One magical moment in the birthing experience is the time directly after birth. As much as possible, I recommend you create a vision of what you want those first hours to look like, and be prepared to seek answers and help in advance to achieve that reality. This includes plans for ensuring skin-to-skin contact, understanding routine interventions and what you want for your baby, having help ready for establishing a breastfeeding relationship, and getting access to donor colostrum if you foresee there will be complications. With a little research and foresight, you may be able to have a birth that exceeds your dreams and that will set your child up for the healthiest possible entrance into her new environment.

"The research is very clear that the optimal birth is a well-supported vaginal birth with the least amount of medical intervention necessary," says Jennifer Block, author of *Pushed: The Painful Truth About Childbirth and Modern Maternity Care*. Natural birth has a variety of interpretations, from unmedicated vaginal birth to just any vaginal birth, regardless of intervention. The research, however, suggests that the definition isn't as far apart as many may think. That's because as soon as one intervention happens, it starts a cascading effect of additional interventions, all of which decrease the chance the women will actually get a vaginal birth. "Many of the routine interventions that are still 'required' in hospital maternity wards across U.S. and Canada, such as continual fetal monitoring, restriction of food and drink, IV fluids, manual rupture of the amniotic sac, Pitocin augmentation, and epidural, are not evidence-based and do not improve outcomes for the baby," says Block.

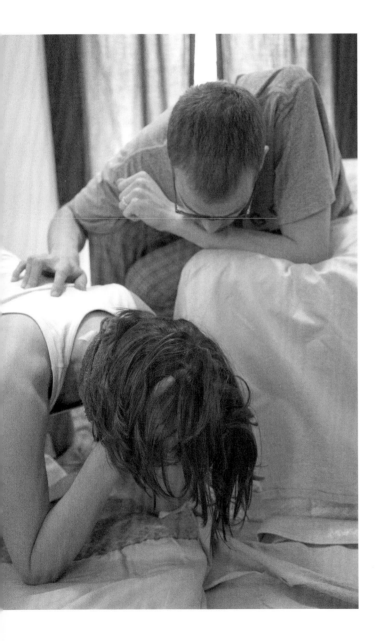

Many women never question these interventions, although they frequently are linked to babies being born by C-section. The FDA has never approved Pitocin (oxytocin) for the use of augmenting labour, and it has been suggested now that mismanagement of Pitocin is the leading cause of liability suits and damage awards in America. Similarly, continuous electronic fetal heart monitoring is another seemingly innocuous medical intervention that studies show may increase the chance of adverse outcomes in a birth. It may not even be particularly effective at reliably indicating fetal distress. What it does do, however, is limit a woman's mobility in labour, which makes it nearly impossible for her to do what her body is telling her to do naturally, which usually involves moving, changing position, and even getting onto her hands and knees. "These interventions often lead down a path toward a Caesarean section, which puts the baby at higher risk for many things, including asthma, gut problems, problems breastfeeding," says Block. At its basis, she says, a C-section is a traumatic birth, just like some vaginal births are traumatic births, and trauma is not a good way to start life or parenting. "Caesarean section is major abdominal surgery and puts a woman at risk for all the complication of surgery, but also future fertility problems, sex problems, and more future Caesareans and greater complications with the next pregnancy, [with] breastfeeding, and a greater chance of hysterectomy. That's why birth matters."

Block says one of the big issues in the United States is that for-profit medicine incentivizes medical intervention. "This puts women right into the middle of a conflict-of-interest in a maternity ward," where the hospital and the physician are motivated to intervene in ways that the woman doesn't want and that aren't in her or the baby's best interest. "Even in Canada and the U.K., Caesarean section rates have been rising in proportion to the U.S. Caesarean section rates." Thus, the problem hasn't been solved even where for-profit medicine isn't the primary factor.

The rise in C-section rates may be just as much about the attitudes of a "new generation of Canadian obstetricians," according to a 2011 *Canadian National Maternity Care Attitudes Survey* that collected information from nearly 70 percent of Canadian obstetricians doing births. The results of this survey were published and revealed, among other results, that the younger generation of obstetricians, defined as under 40, were more likely to favour use of routine epidural, believing it did not interfere with labour, despite evidence to the contrary. Similarly, despite evidence that it is pregnancy itself, not vaginal birth, that results in damage to the pelvic floor, younger obstetricians believed the opposite. They were less supportive of home birth, birth plans, and attempting a vaginal birth after a previous C-section, and they were less interested in peer-reviewed research around birth practices. Perhaps most disturbingly, they were also less likely than their older peers to value the role of maternal choice in the birth process.

"Many women still culturally accept this standard of care, that 'doctor knows best,'" says Block. She explains that in the U.S., there is an open discussion about how refusing to allow women to move freely, eat or drink, try different positions for pushing, or use birth tubs amounts to a type of violence against women. "This goes against medical ethics and a woman's constitutional or charter rights," she says.

When Money Matters More

Physiological birth can have significant cost benefits that are shared by society, but increasing one's chances of getting a natural birth can end up being cost-prohibitive to poor families. An uncomplicated home birth typically costs three to eight thousand dollars, including the prenatal and postnatal care. In a hospital, that amount doubles and usually just covers the birth. A C-section will be more than double an uncomplicated hospital birth. In Canada, most of those costs are covered by our healthcare system (though that system hasn't raised the salaries of midwives in years). Many Canadian families do not have access to midwives, both because of midwife shortages and lack of access in rural communities. Our lower-income communities tend to have more birth interventions and, thus, more complicated and expensive births. In the U.S., many insurance programs will only cover hospital births; thus, a family who wants a home birth will often have to cover the entire cost themselves.

She also says that having a choice of where to birth is very important. "Not only is hospital care largely not evidence-based [as being better] and sometimes downright harmful, it is very expensive. An uncomplicated vaginal birth [in hospital] is three times the cost of a home birth and a Caesarean is four to five times the cost of a home birth, and if there are any complications that require the baby to go to the NICU, multiply that another five times. Midwives as providers and home birth for women who want it make sense for health and economical reasons." She points to a Canadian study that compared birth at home with midwives, birth in a hospital with midwives, and birth in a hospital with a physician. "It showed that women with the best outcomes were the ones that gave birth at home with midwives."

Greening a Hospital Birth

As one midwife said, referring to her three home-birthed children and one hospital-born child, "Homebirth is the Cadillac of birth experiences." Not everyone can have or even wants a Cadillac (personally, I'd prefer a Tesla!), but there are ways to improve the hospital experience. The best is to go in with as much information and support as possible. One thing that will help with both is taking childbirth education classes — Bradley, Lamaze, and Birthing from Within are

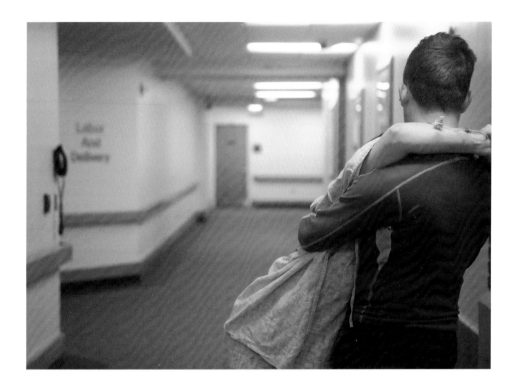

some of the options I'd recommend. And I'd also recommend getting a doula — a person who supports and advocates for the mother through the birth process.

If you will be birthing in the hospital, there are a number of things to consider or plan for after the birth. These include:

- Ensure that your baby can room-in with you and that there is a safe place for the baby to do that. (A hospital bed is not a safe place for co-sleeping.)
- Ask what they do after the baby is born in the case of both a vaginal delivery and a C-section. In either situation, it is ideal to get the baby on the mother as soon as possible, as the physiological benefits to mother and baby of skin-to-skin contact have been well established. And early breastfeeding initiation is essential in helping establish the microbiome and in successfully beginning the breastfeeding relationship.
- Is it a baby-friendly hospital? If not, then ask very specifically how they support the breastfeeding relationship. Make sure they don't insist on giving the baby sugar water or formula if the baby hasn't gained back its birth weight before leaving the hospital or if the baby is a certain size. Most hospitals don't do this anymore because it has been shown to interfere with successful breastfeeding, but some still do.

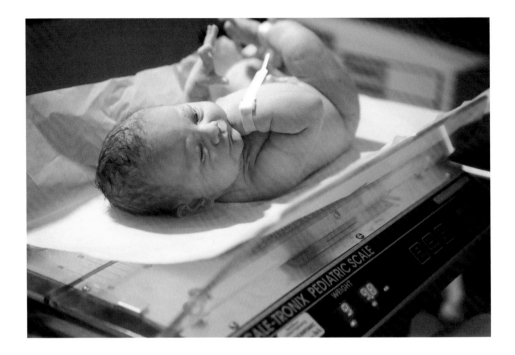

- Will they wait to bathe the baby until after skin-to-skin contact? Skin-to-skin contact immediately is ideal and supported by the research. When they do bathe the baby, can you provide your own bathing items? (The list of ingredients on most hospital products is long and frightening.) Don't forget to include extremely gentle items in your hospital bag.
- Can you keep the placenta in case you want to encapsulate it into postnatal vitamins? According to the midwives with whom I spoke, this is getting increasingly popular, and many hospitals can accommodate the request.
- Will babies who are born by Caesarean section be swabbed with vaginal bacteria? (Read more in **Seeding the Microbiome**, on pages 155–57.)

Preparing for the Sacred Hour After Birth

Skin-to-Skin Contact

What must it be like for the baby entering the world after approximately 266 days in the protective embrace of the womb? In one article on the subject, the doctor writing it said the hour after birth was so important for future outcomes that they called it the "Sacred Hour" at the hospital where she worked. She said, "No one would think of interrupting a wedding ceremony to give the bride and groom details about the flight arrangements for their honeymoon. Everyone recognizes that this information can wait until after the ceremony is completed." Similarly, the research is clear that immediately after labour, a baby needs to be skin-to-skin with her mother if at all possible. It helps the baby stabilize her temperature, breathing, and glucose levels. The baby shows fewer signs of stress. It can help with brain development and facilitate infant self-regulation over time. Mothers also benefit, showing increased confidence in caring for their babies, longer breastfeeding durations, and enhanced maternal behaviours. Indeed, babies can move their way up the body to the breast and self-attach during this skin-to-skin time. I watched both of my babies do it.

Seeding the Microbiome

Just as our understanding of the microbiome is developing as you read this, so is our understanding of how this might be useful in birth. We know, for instance, that "babies delivered by C-section acquire a microbiota that differs from that of vaginally delivered infants, and C-section delivery has been associated with increased risk for immune and metabolic disorders" (*Nature Medicine*, 2016). These disorders include a higher risk of obesity, asthma, and allergies. This study was able to show that babies born via C-section who were swabbed after birth

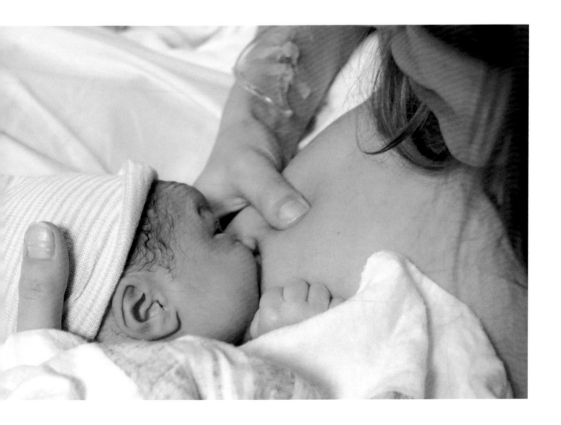

with the mother's vaginal fluids had oral and skin bacterial communities enriched with vaginal bacteria a month later, similar to newborns delivered vaginally, and in contrast to the unexposed C-section babies, who did not have this bacteria. The study does not extend beyond the first 30 days yet, but the lead researcher, Maria G. Dominguez-Bello, believes the differences will continue and is working on a follow-up study that will look at the effects after a year. Indeed, she and others say that the difference in the microbiomes of babies born by C-section (without being "seeded" by vaginal bacteria) and vaginally delivered babies is so great that she can tell even a year after birth which babies were delivered by which method.

The practice of "seeding" babies born via C-section has already entered some hospital practices, but it is far from being routine. Research takes a long time to prove anything, and medicine can take an even longer to adapt to new science. Thus, many hospitals are actively discouraging the practice. They say, rather, to focus on breastfeeding and avoiding unnecessary antibiotics, which are both proven ways to help propagate a baby with necessary and beneficial bacteria. Regardless of how one births, both of these are good practices to focus on.

Not only can antibiotic use after birth affect a baby's microbiome, but animal research suggests that taking antibiotics during pregnancy can both reduce the health and diversity of a mother's bacterial environment and leave the baby, once born, with a lower immunological response and more susceptible to pathogens. This leads to the important issue of antibiotics during labour for Group B strep (GBS). Approximately 10 to 35 percent of pregnant women have GBS, and while it is harmless for most adults, it can cause illness, sometimes severe, in a small percentage of newborn babies. In most parts of Canada, women may choose to test for GBS; then, if they do test positive, they must decide whether to undertake antibiotic therapy during labour, taking into consideration additional risk factors, such as having had a previous baby with GBS disease, having GBS in your actual urine during pregnancy, going into labour at less than 37 weeks, having your water broken for more than 18 hours, or developing a fever during labour. Tests are currently underway to determine whether oral probiotic supplementation may also be effective in treating GBS. Anecdotally, women have treated GBS on their own, prior to labour, but there are obviously no large-scale tests to show this is safe or effective. This self-treatment included taking high-quality probiotics daily, with occasional vaginal use; 2,000 mg a day of vitamin C; daily garlic capsules; and using the garlic-clove-in-the-vagina remedy (described in **The Natural Pregnancy Handbook**) prescribed for yeast infections. Prevention, however, is not much different than what I'd recommend for all pregnant women: eating lots of probiotic-rich fermented food, consuming coconut oil, and eating garlic.

Breast milk is also incredibly effective at seeding the baby's microbiome. The first milk, or the colostrum, contains more than 700 species of microbes. The bacterial makeup of the breast milk changes, so that by six months after birth, more bacterial species associated with healthy mouth areas were present. Studies have also found that not all breast milk is created equal: overweight mothers and mothers who had planned C-sections (though not those who had C-sections after a trial of labour) had less of a diversity of bacteria in their milk. This may suggest that birth hormones play a role in the microbial composition of breast milk. Breastfeeding has been proven to help set up the baby's immune system so that he or she has fewer chronic illnesses later in life.

Vitamin K Shots

One of the first things that will be offered to your baby after birth is a vitamin K shot. As you read in the nutrition chapter, vitamin K is an important nutrient that helps blood to clot. What we also know is that, increasingly, mothers' levels of vitamin K aren't sufficient, and even if they are, it may not adequately pass through the placental barrier and into the baby. If a baby is born with a vitamin K deficiency, they can start to bleed suddenly and severely, and this can even lead to death. Most early cases of deficiency (within the first 24 hours of giving birth) are caused by the mother taking medicines that may interfere with vitamin K, such as the blood thinner warfarin or some anti-seizure medications. Vitamin K is naturally lowest within the seven days after birth. While bleeding problems are most likely during this week, they usually aren't deadly. Vitamin K deficiency–related bleeding can still occur after this, although rarely, and infants with gallbladder disease, cystic fibrosis, or diarrhea, or those who have been given antibiotics may be at greater risk. The vitamin K shot has successfully brought down the number of deaths related to vitamin K deficiency bleeding, although there are also doctors warning that the shot in particular may have unintended risks. There are alternatives, which include oral vitamin K for the baby (which is rarely done in the U.S. because it would mean seeing and dosing the baby at birth, one week, and six weeks old) and supplementing the breastfeeding mother's diet after birth with 2.5 mg of oral vitamin K1 twice a day while seeing the baby routinely to assess efficacy.

Dr. Bethany Hays, functional medicine doctor and obstetrician, says that if a mother is sufficiently nourished and isn't herself at risk for vitamin K deficiency, she wouldn't typically suggest the vitamin K shot. The exception is if the baby is a boy who is being circumcised in the first few days. This is because vitamin K levels remain low until around day eight after birth. Interestingly, in the Jewish tradition, the ceremonial circumcision, or bris, happens on the eighth day of life.

Circumcision

If you have a baby boy, you will be given a choice whether or not to circumcise soon after birth. Increasingly, this is a procedure that more and more people today are opting out of altogether. The AAP and CPS do not consider routine newborn circumcision to be medically necessary. The science that exists shows that there may be a slight decrease in certain communicable diseases, such as HIV, without a foreskin, but it also says that the risk reduction is tiny, mostly only shown in the developing world, and may just be attributed to better hygiene. In other words, for most Canadians there is no medical reason to opt for this elective surgery. If you don't circumcise your son, make sure you teach him how to properly care for his penis. This ought not to be too hard for most women, as taking care of an uncircumcised penis is similar to taking care of a girl's vulva: you don't need to scrub away the white smegma, made up of dead skin cells and oils; don't use harsh soaps; and don't force back the foreskin until it naturally recedes on its own, which can happen anytime from childhood to the teens. After the foreskin recedes on its own, the area under it should be cleaned daily with warm water, just like a vulva.

Successful Breastfeeding

In North America, the majority of mothers want and intend to breastfeed their infants. For those who cannot, there are few losses more deeply felt in the early parenting years. Breastfeeding is at its heart a continuation of the intensely nourishing and profound connection of pregnancy. The deep longing most women feel to breastfeed their babies is backed by the science, which shows that human milk is extremely important for both the baby's and mother's health.

Breastfeeding decreases the incidence of infectious diseases in the breastfed infant, including bacterial meningitis, diarrhea, and infections of the respiratory systems, ears, urinary tract, and gastrointestinal system. Breastfed infants are also less likely to develop allergies, celiac and Crohn's disease, asthma, lymphoma, leukemia, heart disease, high blood pressure, multiple sclerosis, obesity, certain cancers, Hodgkin's disease, and Type 1 and Type 2 diabetes.

Breastfeeding reduces hospital admissions for infants and decreases incidents of sudden infant death syndrome (SIDS). Breastfed babies have higher IQs, and the longer they are breastfed, the greater that IQ gain.

Breastfeeding also has health benefits for the mother, including an association with the decreased incident of breast, ovarian, uterine, and thyroid cancers; osteoporosis; lupus; rheumatoid arthritis; obesity; and postpartum depression. These mothers also have an easier time losing weight postpartum. Some of the data on the benefits of breastfeeding is surprisingly clear: for every year a woman breastfeeds, she reduces her risk of breast cancer by an average of 4.3 percent, according to a meta analysis of 47 international studies on the benefits of breastfeeding published in the *Lancet* in 2002.

The science on breastfeeding is so clear that every major health organization, including the WHO, AAP, and CPS, recommends that women breastfeed for as long as they can, ideally for at least two years, and exclusively for the first six

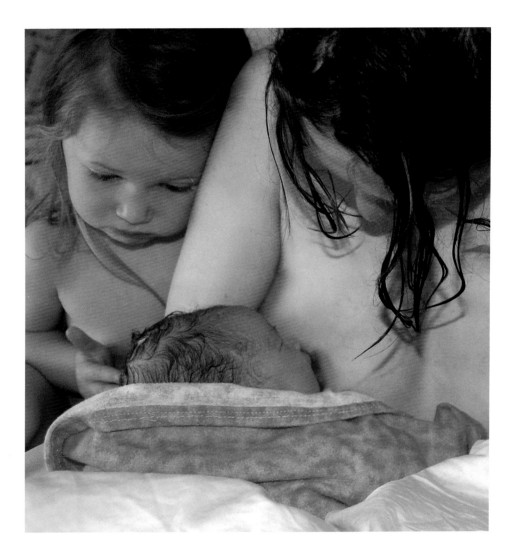

months. Unfortunately, despite 90 percent of mothers wanting to breastfeed, fewer than that number even attempts it in Canada or the United States. Only 26 percent of mothers in Canada and 16 percent in the U.S. make it to the six-month goal of exclusive breastfeeding. B.C. mothers are doing far better than the national average, with 41 percent of mothers succeeding (48 percent on Vancouver Island and 49 percent in and around Vancouver).

The top reason that women gave for stopping breastfeeding was "not enough milk." This despite the fact that very few women — only about 1 to 5 percent — are physiologically incapable of producing milk. When my friend Robin sought out help for poor production, the lactation doctor told her that the greatest indicator that a woman is capable of producing sufficient breast milk is that she produces *any* milk. Usually only rare medical conditions prevent a woman from producing

When Money Matters More

An individual family can save between $700 and $3,000 a year by breast-feeding over buying infant formula. This does not include healthcare savings: babies who don't breastfeed have more doctor visits and respiratory tract infections in the first year than those who are given breast milk. There are studies looking at what countries as a whole could save if the breastfeeding rates were brought just up to the recommended numbers. It's estimated that the U.S. would save at least $3.6 billion in direct benefits. This number doesn't take into account the additional billions that could be saved from less cancer, fewer cases of Type 2 diabetes, and a generally healthier population — just some of the benefits to be gained by breastfeeding. Unfortunately, low-income families who most need these savings are the least likely to breast-feed in both Canada and the United States.

milk at all; some of these conditions include insufficient glandular tissue, breast cancer, hypo-plastic breast syndrome, breast reduction or other extensive breast surgery, or pituitary or thyroid imbalances.

So, if the majority of women in Canada want to nurse and can nurse, what is going wrong that only a quarter of women make it to the six-month goal? The answer may lie in cultural and medical practices. Women in British Columbia don't just happen to have more milk than their eastern counterparts. What they may have, however, is access to support in the form of knowledgeable health care providers, friends and family to help with everything from giving advice on how to make it through those tough first few weeks to holding the baby so the mom can feed herself and nourish her own supply, and jobs that allow women to take a year off to foster the health of their child and themselves.

What we have learned from the countries with the best breastfeeding rates in the developed world, like the Scandinavian nations, is that government policies can and do influence breastfeeding success more than a woman's "supply." These policies include paid parental leave for at least a year, strict limits and guidelines on infant formula advertising and dispersal, and the Baby-Friendly Hospital Initiative. The CDC says, "Hospitals can either help or hinder mothers and babies as they begin to breastfeed," and encourages hospitals to become baby-friendly. Unfortunately, only 12 hospitals or birthing centres in Canada and 170 in the U.S. currently meet the baby-friendly standards. To be designated as "baby-friendly," an institution needs to follow each of the following ten steps for at least 80 percent of all the women and babies it cares for:

1. Have a written breastfeeding policy that is routinely communicated to all health care staff.
2. Train all health care staff in skills necessary to implement the breast-feeding policy.
3. Inform all pregnant women about the benefits and management of breastfeeding.
4. Help mothers initiate breastfeeding within a half hour after birth.
5. Show mothers how to breastfeed and maintain lactation even when they are separated from their infants.
6. Give newborns no food or drink other than breast milk, unless medically indicated.
7. Practise rooming-in: allow mothers and infants to remain together 24 hours a day.
8. Encourage breastfeeding on demand.
9. Give no artificial teats or pacifiers (also called dummies or soothers) to breastfeeding infants.
10. Foster the establishment of breastfeeding support groups and refer mothers to them at discharge from the hospital or clinic.

The Breastfeeding Breakdown

In my experience, if the breastfeeding relationship is going to break down, it does so in the first 12 weeks. Usually, it is due to a combination of bad medical advice and lack of support. Doctors who aren't familiar with the benefits of breastfeeding babies can be the biggest hindrance. While I was writing this chapter, my sister called in tears because her baby had jaundice and the doctor advised her to supplement with infant formula. This was my sister's third baby, so she knew enough to seek out a second opinion, and what she discovered was that this old advice was no longer the recommended course of action in her case. Luckily, she persevered and nursed the baby more, and he was down to normal bilirubin levels the very next day. By the time her two-week appointment arrived, the baby hadn't quite gained back his birth weight. Again, the doctor advised that my sister supplement with formula. A full-term, full-weight baby who is breastfed may take two weeks to gain back birth weight, but any longer is usually a sign that something needs help in the breastfeeding relationship. Is it latch? Is it supply? Or do the woman and baby just need a bit more time? A doctor who isn't familiar with breastfeeding babies is not likely to have the answers or know that, for example, a breastfed baby routinely has higher bilirubin levels and follows a different growth chart than an infant who has not been breastfed. In my sister's case, the doctor wasn't even able to refer her somewhere for lactation support. My sister, luckily, found her way to a lactation consultant, who said that everything looked great and gave my sister

When Money Matters More

There are a number of assistance programs in the United States to help poorer families, including Women, Infants and Children (WIC). WIC calculates that it costs about 45 percent less to support a breastfeeding mother than a formula-feeding mother. The U.S. spends $578 million in federal funds every year to buy formula for babies. My sister was able to get lactation support, regular weigh-ins for her baby, and help finding a breastfeeding support group through her local WIC office. In Canada, there is a noted gap in availability of postpartum care, particularly in relation to breastfeeding support, based on income. Quebec is currently the only province in Canada that gives a specific monthly breastfeeding allowance to women on public assistance with new babies who are breastfeeding. The La Leche League is one of the best sources of free lactation support in both the U.S. (www.lllusa.org) and Canada (www.lllc.ca).

some additional tips on draining the breasts and keeping the baby awake for more thorough feedings. Her son met his weight goals by three weeks and is now a chubby, happy, and exclusively breastfed five-month-old baby.

A woman who hasn't breastfed before may not know that it can take up to a week for the milk to come in, that it takes (sometimes difficult) practice to develop a good latch, and that it gets easier (even enjoyable) over time. Even if she has "read up" on it, like I did, "women don't give birth or breastfeed in their brains," says Dr. Hays. Women often need a more physical, tangible kind of help. Some doctors are great at this. I was lucky enough to have both midwives and a family doctor with my first baby, all of whom were extremely knowledgeable about breastfeeding and breastfed babies. They were able to help me with my latch, correct small early issues, and refer me to additional breastfeeding support. As the baby-friendly hospital guidelines show, it is essential for a new breastfeeding mom to have someone she trusts to say "it's okay" and help her make it so. Sometimes it's not a healthcare provider, but a lactation consultant, support group, or wise friend. Social media can be a great way to find a breastfeeding peer group near you. La Leche League offers free peer support at **1-877-4-LALECHE** (1-877-452-5324) in the U.S. or **1-800-665-4324** in Canada, or you can visit them online at www.lllusa.org (U.S.) and www.lllc.ca (Canada).

Even when a woman has previous experience, breastfeeding can be hard. My second baby was tongue-tied. She didn't have a severe case, but she did have the telltale heart-shaped tongue. I could tell something wasn't quite right, because nursing hurt so much more with her than it had with the first, but I grinned and bore it instead of getting her frenulum (the bit of tissue that connects the bottom of the tongue to the floor of the mouth) snipped. Eventually it loosened on its own and breastfeeding felt normal, but it took more than six months. Another friend had a similar situation but had to leave the hospital where she had given birth and travel to the far end of her city to find a doctor who could snip the baby's frenulum. Another friend suffered on for six weeks and nearly gave up nursing from the pain, until she finally figured it out and had her baby's frenulum snipped, only to instantly discover that nursing could be enjoyable. After almost stopping at six weeks, she went on to nurse her child for two years.

Similarly, I've known mothers who had those severe medical conditions that make it almost impossible to produce enough milk. These mothers were intent on providing breast milk to their babies and were able to do so. One of the tools that can help in cases of low supply is a supplemental nursing system, which is a feeding tube that attaches a bottle (with the supplemented milk) to the mother's actual breast so that the baby is still suckling and stimulating the mothers supply and practising good latch while getting additional food. In a couple of the cases the women also chose to use pharmaceutical support in the form of domperidone, which is not currently approved for the use of stimulating milk production in Canada but is considered by many to be the safest available pharmaceutical, especially in that it doesn't pass through the blood-brain barrier.

If you are worried about over-the-counter or prescription drug use or alcohol while breastfeeding, you will be happy to know that in almost all cases there are safer drugs available for the breastfeeding mother. For many drugs, including cigarettes and alcohol, women are still advised to breastfeed, but to wait for the drugs to leave their system. Learn more about the safety of specific drugs at Motherisk, the U.S. National Library of Medicine's LactMed website, or Dr. Hale's InfantRisk website. (See the **Further Reading** section for contact information.)

Healthy Feeding Options When Not Breastfeeding

Some mothers also take part in breast milk sharing. This idea used to be quite common in the years before the invention of infant formulas. Indeed, upper class women would often hire a wet nurse specifically so they didn't have to be tied to breastfeeding the babies themselves; it was known even then that babies who were breastfed did better than those who were given milk from other animals. This trend may be coming back. The United Arab Emirates (UAE) passed a clause mandating women breastfeed their babies for two years as part of their new Child Rights Law. Despite the obvious concerns with such a law, it also includes the recognition that, even in the developed world, not being breastfed doubles an infant's chance of neonatal death. It also promised a government-funded wet nurse for those mothers who couldn't breastfeed.

When Money Matters More

One of the issues that clearly affect breastfeeding rates in both Canada and the United States is access to paid maternity leave. The Family Leave and Medical Act in the U.S. requires that employers of a certain size offer 12 weeks of unpaid leave after the birth of a child for women employed for at least a year before the birth (and with a minimum of 1,250 hours worked in that year). That makes the U.S. the only developed country with no paid maternity leave. Canada generally provides 15 weeks of paid maternity leave at up to 55 percent of a woman's wages, as long as she was employed for at least a year before the birth of the child and had worked at least 600 hours. By combining maternity leave, parental benefits, and sick leave, a woman could take up to 50 weeks of parental leave (maximum pay just over $400/week), with some of this time able to be split with the father or partner. There are significant differences in leave opportunities between the Canadian provinces, with Quebec in particular standing out with a program that covers parents at a higher rate of pay for maternity leave and includes benefits for those who were self-employed or only partially employed. They also provide a five-week, 70-percent-paid paternity leave. Low-income women in Canada often do not qualify for paid parental leave.

In many cases, women in the U.S. and Canada are left to figure out on their own how to get the care they need to support healthy births and postpartum periods. There are resources available to help. If you are on public assistance in Canada and wonder what your province provides, visit the Public Health Agency of Canada's website at www.phac-aspc.gc.ca/hp-gs/prov-eng.php.

The UAE isn't the only place that breast milk is being given a value. In North America, women (and others) can buy and sell breast milk online. Some are doing this on websites like www.craigslist.com, while others are doing it through businesses like www.onlythebreast.com, where milk seems to go for an average of US$2 an ounce, plus shipping. For those who like to go local and meet their milk supplier, there are a number of organizations using social media to help connect babies-in-need with donors of free breast milk. These include Human Milk 4 Human Babies, which promotes "informed milk-sharing" and is online at www.hm4hb.net, and Eats on Feets, which believes "community-based milk

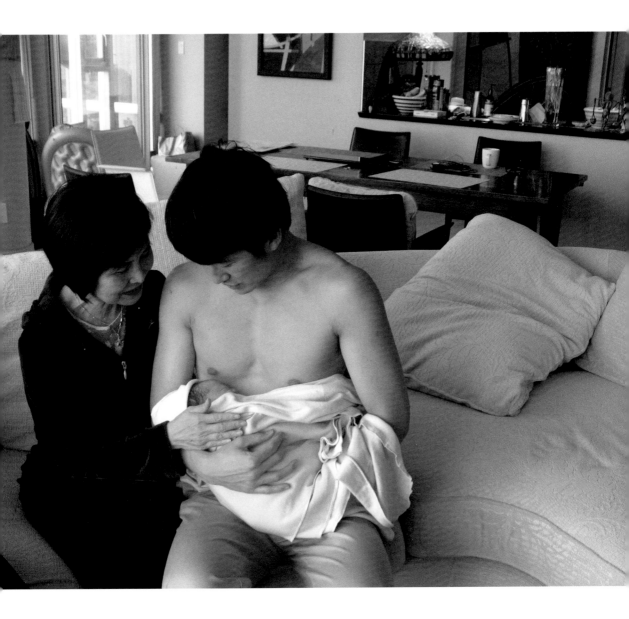

sharing is normal" and can be found online at www.eatsonfeets.org. They developed the Four Pillars of Safe Breast Milk Sharing: informed choice, donor screening, safe handling, and options for home pasteurization. I was lucky enough to be able to donate breast milk to a friend with my first child. I'm still in awe of how she managed to exclusively breastfeed her baby, despite a medical condition limiting her own supply, for her child's first six months, and this was before the advent of social media to help. I've been similarly impressed by the many adoptive parents I have met who similarly made use of milk banks, community resources, and family to get breast milk to their babies.

The research shows that women with supportive partners are twice as likely to successfully meet their breastfeeding goals. It really does take a village. Partners can help by being on nighttime changing duty, bringing and taking the child from the mother to nurse, helping with pumping, and, once the latch and breastfeeding relationship is well established, even giving the baby bottles of breast milk. When a mother isn't able to nurse herself, the partner can help by researching viable options, arranging breast milk donations, and helping feed the baby. You don't need breasts to "nurse" a baby, who benefits from cuddling, eye contact, and loving connections. So, never prop the bottle up and just leave a young baby to feed himself; let eating be communal right from the beginning.

When Breast Milk Isn't an Option

If you are going to use formula, there are a few things you need to know. First, it's possible and healthier to make your own. When my husband was a baby, he was given homemade goat milk formula. You can get excellent time-tested advice and research about making your own infant formula from the Weston A. Price Foundation and from the book *Nourishing Traditions* by Sally Fallon Morell. The basic recipe includes whole milk, whey, lactose, Bifidobacterium infantis, cream, cod liver oil, unrefined sunflower oil, extra-virgin olive oil, coconut oil, nutritional yeast, gelatin, and acerola powder. There is also a goat milk recipe that is basically just organic raw goat milk with the addition of nutritional yeast and pureed frozen, organic, raw chicken liver. Both sources also offer a stock-based formula made with beef or chicken bones that is suitable for babies who can't handle much cow protein. There are also ideas for supplementing your organic commercial infant formula with items like egg yolks and cod liver oil to make it easier to digest and healthier.

If buying commercial infant formula, I strongly suggest you only **buy it powdered and organic**. Unfortunately, most organic infant formula brands don't actually meet the organic standards set up in North America and contain ingredients banned in infant formulas in the EU.

A better organic commercial formula may be an organic one from Europe, such as Holle from Germany. In North America, Baby's Only, which is marketed for toddlers though it is appropriate for younger babies as well, has some advantages over the other commercial formulas. It comes in a BPA-free can, is one of the only commercial formulas that doesn't contain hexane-derived DHA/ARA, and was the first to eliminate arsenic (found in almost all commercially grown rice) from its infant formula.

Soy formula should be avoided due to its ability to harm a developing endocrine system and mimic estrogen, as well as its potentially dangerous levels of aluminum and manganese. It has been suggested that soy-based infant formula may be linked to ADHD, early onset of menses, and early formation of breast tissue. Most major health organizations in both Canada and the U.S. recommend against using soy formula unless it is medically necessary, which is rare.

Always use clean, filtered water to mix with your powdered baby formula, or when the child is older and you are giving straight water. Even in North America, tap water and bottled water can be sources of parasites and bacteria, as well as numerous other contaminants and pesticides. Exclusively breastfed babies do not need additional water supplementation.

Whatever you feed your baby, if you supplement or just want a night off from breastfeeding, you may want bottles. Glass or stainless steel options are the safest and are also easy to maintain. Avoid using plastic bottles, even those labelled BPA-free, almost all of which still contain endocrine disruptors. Babies can be taught to drink out of a cup from a very young age, and thus you can avoid baby bottles altogether if you are so motivated.

How to Have a Green Birth and Beyond: Checklist

The research is clear: women who take an active role in planning for their births are more likely to be satisfied with their birth experiences. Whether a woman chooses to have her baby in a hospital, in a birth centre, or at home, there is some work and advance planning she has to do to ensure she is getting what she wants and expects. Here are a series of action steps listed from ♥♥♥ (biggest impact, and possibly more work) to ♥ (quick and easy) to help your green your birth experience and beyond.

1. ♥♥♥ **Interview care providers.** Come on ladies: we try out a car before we buy it, we interview nannies, and we even read online reviews of restaurants and salons before we visit, so why would we not interview the care providers we expect to attend our births? Remember, many obstetricians/gynecologists are *not* trained in "normal" births, but are specialists in what can go wrong. In B.C., most babies are delivered by family doctors or midwives. In the U.S., most women just go to the OB/GYN she has always gone to. If you want a vaginal birth, I strongly encourage you to include midwives in your interview process (and family doctors when midwives aren't feasible).

2. ♥♥ **Ask meaningful questions.** Like many women, it is hard for me to ask questions of authority figures, especially if I think the person won't like my questions. Ask anyway! In the hospital on the day of your delivery is too late. (It is also probably too late at 36 weeks, so start right away.) At a minimum, I suggest you ask the following:

   • What is the care provider's rate of Caesarean section for their practice and at the hospital where they work, if applicable?

- What is the rate of episiotomy? Routine episiotomy use is not supported by research, and a doctor's rate should be below 15 percent.
- What does the doctor or midwife do during a birth to help prevent tearing?
- Will you be allowed to labour or birth in water, such as in a shower or birthing tub? Water is considered a safe and effective method of pain management in labour and can help prevent tearing during pushing.

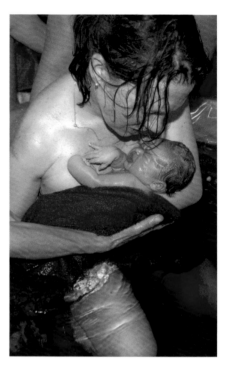

- What support does the midwife or doctor provide to help with pain relief, other than drugs? (See below for the list of the six comfort practices that promote a healthy birth.)
- What is the rate of epidural? When are most epidurals started, if used? Epidurals have been linked with an increased chance of maternal fever, the need for vacuum extraction or forceps, serious perineal tears, and many other labour interventions, including C-section. High epidural rates may suggest the practice doesn't provide more natural support. At the very least, I suggest you try to delay the epidural for as long as possible.
- Who is most likely to attend your baby's delivery? Is it an individual or group practice? If it's a group practice, will you have any say in who attends? How many other labouring women will the doctor, midwife, or nurse usually be responsible for at the same time?
- How does your care provider define "high-risk"? Different practitioners will have different answers. For instance, some doctors will consider you high-risk if you have had a previous C-section, and they will want to schedule your next Caesarean delivery, while other practitioners will allow you to try for a vaginal birth after Caesarean (VBAC). Similarly, some practitioners consider it fine to go two weeks past your estimated due date, while others will want to induce you if you are less than a week past. (Induction could double your risk of having to undergo a C-section.)
- How will the baby be monitored during labour? Continual electronic fetal monitoring (EFM) is often used in hospitals, but is not linked with improved outcomes. When a woman gets continual EFM, it restricts her ability to be active and move around during labour and makes it unlikely that she can use

Perineal Massage

The perineum is the soft skin between the vulva and the anus. This area receives pressure during pushing and can tear, and it is especially vulnerable during a woman's first birth. Tears can range from small, natural tears that will heal on their own or with the help of just a stitch or two. Others can be severe, tearing through multiple layers of the skin, and take stitches and a great deal more time to heal. There are some things that have been shown to help reduce the risk of tearing, and they include a diet rich in healthy fats and other foods good for the skin (see tips on preventing stretch marks on page 103 of **The Natural Pregnancy Handbook**), water birth, foregoing directed pushing and episiotomy and epidurals, and the use of perineal massage starting at approximately 34 weeks. Midwife Kate Koyote says that another benefit of perineal massage is that it helps women learn to relax into the intense stretching sensation associated with the pushing stage, a practice that is of great help during natural labour.

Technique: Start with clean hands (yours or a partner's) and nails trimmed, food grade oil nearby (I suggest olive oil, jojoba oil, or cocoa butter), and a relaxed perineum — a warm bath or washcloth compress can help with this. Get comfortable. Apply oil to your fingers and perineum. Insert two fingers or your thumbs into your vagina. Gently and firmly apply pressure toward your anus and pull the fingers apart at the same time so that the stretch is both downward and outward. Only stretch to the point of a stretching sensation. It should not hurt or burn. Breathe and relax. Continue around your perineum, so the points of pressure circle around like the hours on a clock face. Ten minutes of practice is plenty. Breathe and relax into the stretch the entire time; remember that the point is to practise relaxing into the stretching sensation, not to achieve a certain amount of actual stretching.

water for pain relief. Alternatively, monitoring with a doppler or fetoscope are safe and effective options that allow for freedom of movement.

- Will you be allowed and encouraged to move during labour, eat and drink, and try out different positions for the birth? Research supports mother's being free to move during labour, to drink when thirsty, and eat lightly if interested. The research also suggests avoiding back-lying positions for pushing.

3. ♥♥ **Know the six comfort practices that promote healthy birth.** Make sure you are realistically in a situation where you can get all six (or as many as you want). They are

- let labour begin on its own;
- walk, move around, and change position throughout labour;
- bring a loved one, friend, or doula for continuous support;
- avoid any intervention that isn't medically necessary;
- avoid giving birth on your back, and follow your body's urges; and
- keep mother and baby together.

4. ♥♥ **Remember, you are not likely to be the exception.** Plan as if the statistics do apply to you: if a doctor has a 55 percent C-section rate, that means there's a good chance you might end up with a C-section. If this is your first baby, it is particularly important to consider what the impact of subtle (or not so subtle) pressure from your caregiver might be in influencing your birth experience. Save the positive thinking for the birth and plan based on the facts.

5. ♥♥ **Consider childbirth education classes.** It is best to find a class or group that isn't affiliated with a hospital so that you will get information that is unbiased and does more than just prepare you for an epidural. Bradley, Lamaze, and Birthing from Within are all widely available options.

6. ♥♥ **Watch and read about real (especially positive) birth experiences.** Birth is *nothing* like what you see on TV (with the water breaking, a bunch of screaming and cursing, and a baby delivered before the next commercial). You can watch natural birth videos (rent them, or borrow them from your local library or midwife practice, or find them on YouTube), read books, and talk to your friends. These more gentle videos and books are a great way to prepare older siblings for a birth as well. My daughter would routinely remind me in the days before my birth to practise the gentle moaning and pelvic circles we saw in one such video.

7. ♥♥ **If you want a vaginal birth after previously having had a Caesarean (VBAC),** start asking questions and interviewing caregivers early. Despite a growing body of evidence to show that VBACs are the preferred option for most women and are associated with better outcomes both in current and future pregnancies, many hospitals and providers still won't allow them or aren't prepared to really support a trial of labour after a previous C-section. Learn more about VBAC at the International Cesarean Awareness Network (www.ican-online.org).

Placental Encapsulation

"We are one of the only mammals that don't eat our own placentas," says the midwife Kate Koyote. If your immediate thought is yuck, don't worry. Now there is placental encapsulation, where the placenta is freeze-dried and encapsulated into a postpartum vitamin. (This seems far better than keeping your placenta in your freezer until the day before Christmas, when your entire family is about to move, forever, to another country, and then wondering "What do I do with it?" while looking forlornly at the frozen soil. Sorry, neighbours!)

The idea is that a woman's own placenta can replenish some of the hormones and vital nutrients necessary for postpartum health. While there haven't been huge double-blind studies, they are underway, and early research suggests that it doesn't do harm and may help with milk supply and baby weight gain, and may even ward off postpartum depression. It isn't, however, a significant source of iron, so while the early anecdotal evidence is good, it may not be a panacea of all nutritional needs. In other words, you may need to pop your placental pill and still sit down to a steak. If you are interested in placental encapsulation, plan in advance! There are services popping up all over the world that will come and pick up your placenta from home or hospital (and help you preserve it correctly until they get there) and then bring it back in pill form. If you can't find or afford placental encapsulation (it often runs $200 to $400 for the service), lots of women find another way to eat their placenta. Red smoothie, anyone? But seriously, you can cut away the membranes and blend the placenta in with a smoothie or cook it up like meat to eat with spaghetti sauce or in a stew. Seriously, you really can.

8. ♥♥ **If you are birthing at a hospital**, or if the hospital is only the back-up plan, find out what the hospital policies are for the time immediately after birth, including:

- Will you be able to have the baby skin-to-skin after birth?
- Will they wait to clamp the cord?
- Will they wait to do measurements for at least an hour?
- Will you be able to provide your own soaps for the baby?

- Will you be able to keep the placenta?
- Will you be able to room with the baby and provide a safe co-sleeping bed for the baby?

If you end up having to undergo a C-section, will you still be able to keep the baby with you afterward, get skin-to-skin, and keep the placenta? Will they facilitate a vaginal flora swap?

9. ♥♥ **Have a plan for getting your baby breast milk.** Will you breast-feed? Who can help if things go wrong? Keep the numbers of a lactation consultant and a knowledgeable friend nearby. If you aren't breastfeeding, is there any way you can get your baby colostrum? This first milk that a woman produces is so high in nutrients, necessary microbes, and anti-bodies that the WHO refers to it as the baby's "first immunization." Can your midwife, doctor, or a breast milk sharing group help you gain access to a trustworthy source of colostrum? Will you be able to find a breast milk donor for longer, or will you make your own formula or buy a better commercially available option? Figuring this out and preparing before the birth will help you make a healthy decision and be able to execute it.

10. ♥ **Do your research and get informed.** Check out the end of this book for great additional reading material.

The Prenatal Yoga Handbook

• •

The practice of prenatal yoga is an opportunity to train both the body and the mind to ease pregnancy symptoms and prepare for birth and parenthood. "In pregnancy a woman must be both strong and soft," says Insiya Rasiwala-Finn, an internationally recognized yoga teacher, a mama, and the writer and publisher of the website www.yogue.ca. Rasiwala-Finn, a Canadian originally from India, is passionate about taking the wisdom traditions of yoga and Ayurveda (a form of alternative medicine with its roots in India) and applying them to modern life. She says that in Ayurvedic terms, women "become more Kapha during pregnancy, more fluid. You slow down and walk differently." She says that for women who fight these changes, it can make them "more anxious and jittery. It can interfere with the hormonal balance and the growth of the baby." She recommends meditation, mindfulness, and yoga to help women "inhabit the pregnancy in harmony with nature."

"Excellent prenatal yoga teachers help their students have a real experience of how to live more enjoyably off the mat, integrating yoga into every moment of their lives," says Cassandra Rodgers, co-founder of Amala School of Prenatal Yoga in Chicago. She encourages women to look for prenatal yoga teachers through the Yoga Alliance (RPYS).

Her school trains yoga teachers and women's health professionals to provide pregnant women with supportive and empowering classes that help them embrace the changes of pregnancy, prepare for giving birth, and find postpartum community. Find certified teachers and learn more at www.amalaprenatalyoga.com.

The 20-Minute Prenatal Yoga Sequence

It's important to remember that any exercise during pregnancy ought to be gentle and careful and avoided during times of pain or acute discomfort. Let the focus of your yoga practice be mindfulness: noticing the new sensations of a growing body and brain. "Less is more," says Rodgers. "You are already 'doing' when you are standing still." The body is loaded with relaxin during pregnancy, and as I learned the hard way, over-stretching can result in injuries that will last many years after; instead, focus on strength, stability, and making "space" for the baby. Remember to be very slow to transition between poses and listen to your body.

Seated Bound Angle

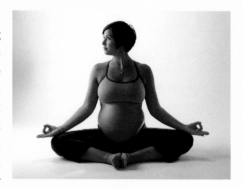

Sit on a folded blanket so the sitting bones are supported but the legs come off. Press the sitting bones down into the blanket as the spine lifts up. Press the outer edges of the feet together and extend the inner thighs away toward the knees. Breathe. Focus on creating space through the abdominal area rather than stretching. Don't overdo it. Consider putting blocks, pillows, or blankets under the knees for support.

Table Pose to Cat and Cow (with Optional Leg Extension and Hip Circles)

These are great warm-up poses that can be done every day and will help keep the spine and pelvis supple and aligned.

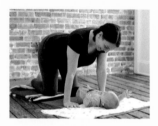 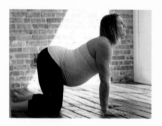 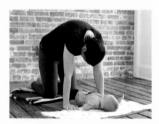

Start on all fours with palms and tops of feet on mat, and with wrists under shoulders and knees under hips. This is table pose. On inhale, look up, stretching through head and hips, letting the back of the shoulders come firmly forward into the spine and allowing the belly to gently release toward the earth. This is cow pose. On the exhale, look down, visualize the navel moving gently toward the spine as you drop the head and round the back into cat pose.

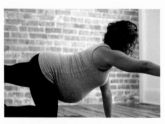

If this feels great, you can work on greater balancing by extending the opposite arm and leg away from each other. Reach out the hand and the leg, feeling the strength that comes from the opposing resistance. Do both sides.

From table pose, you can also rotate the hips in circles. Imagine you are drawing a circle on the floor below you and draw the circle to the left and the right.

Supported Child's Pose

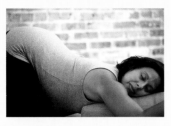

Child's pose is done sitting on the shins with the tops of the feet on the ground. The hips will extend toward the heels and the crown of the head stretches forward in the opposite direction. When pregnant, make sure the knees are wider than the torso and that you have a bolster, blankets, or pillows under your chest as high as needed to make room for the belly. The overall idea of this pose is one of relaxation and letting go.

Downward-Facing Dog

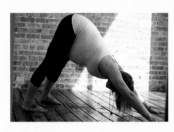

From the table pose, transition into the downward dog pose by pressing the hands into the floor and the heels toward the floor, moving the hips up and away from both. This pose stretches the legs, releases the weight on the spine, and opens the hips. Keep the feet really wide. If this is too intense or your belly is in the way, do the same pose with your hands on a chair stabilized against the wall or just press the hands directly into the wall at hip-level, making a 45-degree angle. Hold the pose for three breaths and slowly come down from the pose the same way you came into it.

Warrior Two

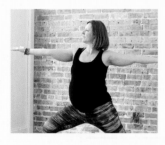

Stand with legs wide and feet firmly planted so that the left foot is forward with toes just a bit turned in, while the toes of the right foot are perpendicular to the body. The hips are mostly squared forward directly under the shoulders. Keep the left leg long and straight while the right leg bends to a square over the right foot. Don't extend the knee beyond the right foot. Press both feet down and lift both sides of the torso up evenly. Extend the arms. Hold for a couple of breaths, and then do the other side.

Goddess

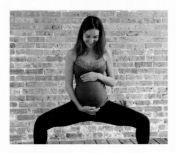

Stand with legs wide and feet firmly planted, but with toes pointed away from each other. Press the legs down and bend the knees so that the knee extends in line with the feet but not beyond. Press down through the feet and stretch up through the torso, keeping both sides pressing and stretching equally.

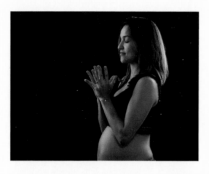

Tadasana

Stand upright and firmly on both feet, spreading the feet wide and firmly planting into the ground. Press the feet down and move the knee caps upward, let the hips move down and the head lift upward. Focus on extending the left and right side of the torso evenly to make room for the growing baby. Breathe.

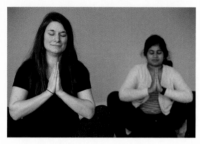

Seated Squat

From standing, have the feet wide and turned outward. Sit down into a squat on a block, bolster, or blankets (you can also do without the props if you feel okay without the support). Let the sitting bones drop down, and at the same time lift up through the torso and crown of the head. Allow the elbows to rest inside the knees, and press out as the knees also hug into the elbows, creating some resistance, both stretching and stabilizing.

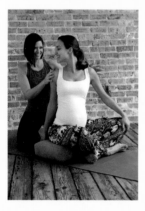

Seated Twist

Sit on a bolster or chair, both sitting bones pressing firmly into the seat and crown of the head stretching up. Reach the right arm behind you and press down into the floor, bolster, or chair, keep the torso lifting up. Place the left hand against the inside of the left leg and press against the leg, while the leg stays firm, to assist the twist. Keep the twist gentle and focus on lifting evenly through the sides of the torso. Take a couple of breaths and return to the centre for a breath, then do the same on the left.

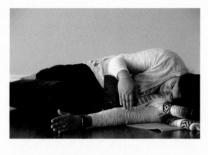

Side-Lying Savasana (for Later Pregnancy)

Savasana, which is the ultimate resting pose in yoga, when done with support, is great in later pregnancy both to relax after a yoga practice and to help position the baby for birth. Lie on the left side with the right leg and right arm supported by a bolster, pillows, or blankets. Have a pillow under the head as well. Let your entire body relax into this pose. Stay as long as you can.

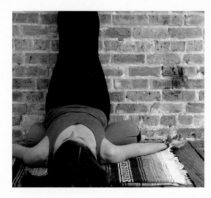

Legs Up the Wall (for Early Pregnancy and Postpartum)

This pose is great for conception, early pregnancy, and the postpartum period, but is best avoided during the third trimester. It helps calm the mind and increases circulation. The only trick is getting into the pose. Have a bolster or a few folded blankets near the wall to support your sacrum (the large, triangular bone at the base of the spine). Once there, extend your legs up the wall, pressing through the feet to extend the legs while resting the sacrum on the bolster. Release the arms beside the torso. This is a great time for an eye pillow. Breathe. Feel the stability of the earth underneath you. Feel the life growing within. Feel your body making space. From this place, you can practise belly breathing.

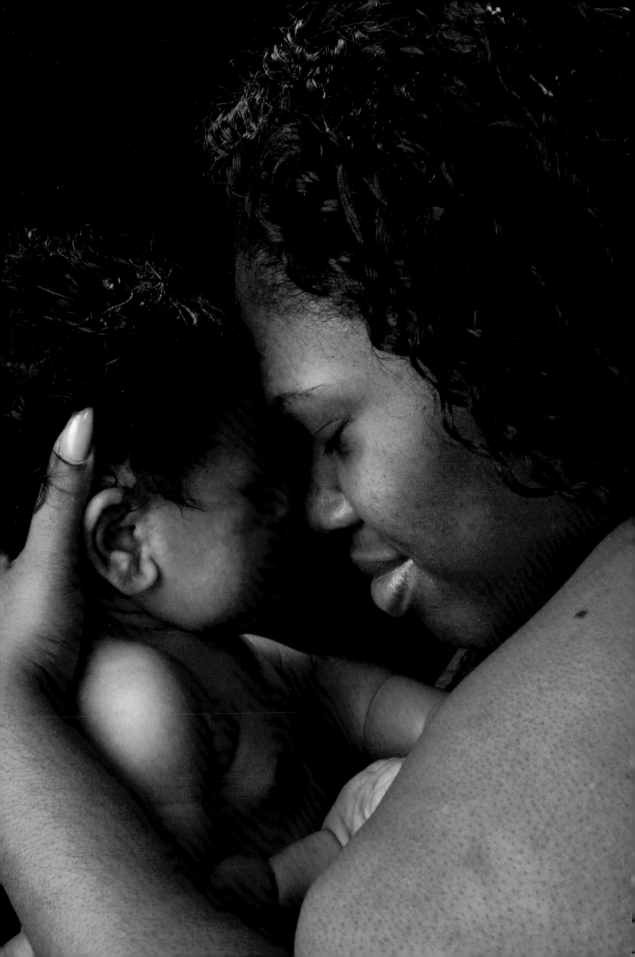

chapter seven

Greening the Fourth Trimester and Preparing for Postpartum Bliss

• •

I remember the day after having my first child. It was a bright, cold November morning and I was astonished because, after sleeping for about eight hours straight, my new baby woke up howling. It felt like she continued screaming for the next two years. It was as shocking as that point in labour when I realized I had to push *while* I had contractions. I swear, in the 200 books I had read about birth, they didn't mention that. They didn't seem to mention the day after the birth either.

Pregnancy is depleting work, regardless of how easy or difficult it is, but birth is hard, exhausting work that leaves your body and mind tapped. Then, suddenly, you must recover, learn how to do physically challenging new things (like breastfeeding), and figure out how to care for a new life, all on shockingly little sleep and with a baby who cries, or in my case howls, a lot of the time. It's not an easy time for many people.

"Don't have too many visitors in the first week after having a baby," cautions midwife Kate Koyote. "Allow yourself the space that you need to bond with the baby and to create that sacred space to allow everything else that needs to happen in that period to happen." In her busy practice, she says that those who have too many visitors have a rockier start. It can be even more work to protect a mother's space in the hospital: "There are bells ringing, nurses coming in to check, the mother-in-law says one thing, and the midwife something else, and it can be hard for the mother to hear for herself what is needed."

It was during the period after birth when I was most thankful for my home births: sleeping in my own bed, waking to a house that the midwives had left clean, and having the midwives come to me the next day and for every other appointment for the six weeks after — it felt great. Or, rather, it felt just barely manageable. I can't imagine how I would have gotten in a car or on the bus to get home or take my baby, say, across the city to a doctor's appointment.

Regardless of where your baby is born, there is a great deal you can do to plan for success in the first weeks after birth. "Women need to have lined up these things *before* giving birth. They have no idea how tired they are going to be, how all of the sudden their day is gone: 75 percent of it may have been spent staring at their baby. They aren't going to be searching online to see who does placenta encapsulation," cautions Koyote.

The Research

The Fourth Trimester refers to the three to six months after birth when the baby is still so vulnerable and, well, unformed. A newborn is more like a fetus than an older child and benefits from more womb-like care for these first few months of life. The science backs up this idea: the blood-brain barrier doesn't fully develop until around six months, the organs of detoxification continue to develop during the first year, massive neurological development continues for the first couple of years, and the immune system similarly takes years to fully form. Babies who are able to safely bond to a primary caregiver, given lots of time for rest and skin-to-skin snuggling, and protected from overstimulation and toxin exposure go on to be healthier children and adults. This concept is at the basis of why so many countries offer paid maternity and paternity leave: we all do better when our children do better. Unfortunately, in North America, parents too often find themselves on their own trying to figure out how to "do better." In many ways, simplicity is the key, and achieving it takes a lot of planning for most of us.

What Is Stress?

I have always hated when someone reminded me to "stop stressing." I find it literally stressful to hear, and even more so knowing that too much stress is toxic. I have always appreciated those studies that show a little bit of stress can be beneficial to your health. Yet, that's the point; it's no longer a little bit of stress. One book on the subject estimates that our daily stress is one hundred times greater today than that faced by our grandparents. And our babies are being influenced by our feelings of stress even while in the womb, especially for girls-to-be, who are particularly vulnerable to their mother's stress while in utero.

"For many women it's go go go from the morning when they wake up until they go to bed; it's fast food, fast internet, fast everything, and I think that combines to create unusual stress on the organism," says obstetrician Dr. Bethany Hays. Stress is a term that was coined by the Canadian endocrinologist Hans Selye. It's generally referred to as the "internal or external pressures on an organism that it must respond to in order to function and stay alive."

There is the strain of the outside influence, and then there is the body's response to it. The cells in your body can't tell the difference between the thought "there is a sabretooth tiger at the door of the cave" and "the taxman is coming on the fifteenth." Either way, the body gets the same signals, explains Hays, and responds with the same mechanisms it did in the caveman era: fight, flee, or freeze. Your adrenal and cortisol (and ultimately insulin) levels go up, "which makes vision and hearing sharper, restricts blood vessels and moves the blood to muscles so you can run away, and activates the prefrontal cortex so you can figure out how to get away."

As the adrenal levels go up, so do cortisol levels. It raises your blood sugar so that there is enough sugar in the muscles and turns off any competing high-energy symptoms, such as your immune system, reproductive system, and memory, "because you don't need these to get away from the tiger," says Hays. If you don't immediately make use of that extra sugar by running away from the tiger (or the tax man), then your body stores it, which raises insulin levels.

Insulin helps get rid of sugar, but it also is a growth hormone. If you are grown already, your cells don't need that insulin so they ignore it, a situation which can lead to insulin resistance or Type 2 diabetes. Hays says it's typical in our culture to see people in their twenties and thirties being go-go-go. They are accustomed to high adrenaline with their corresponding body type of muscular legs and skinny arms. These same people in their thirties and forties end up with high cortisol levels and have stored fat around the middle and poor memories. Then in their fifties and sixties they have high insulin, which results in them putting on weight everywhere and being carted in wheelchairs because of inflammation.

"Stress is a response to high adrenaline; it can be internal and external, imagined or real, constant and low or immediate and very high. The immediate, very high we can handle. The repeated high level or constant low level is what tends to get us in trouble." Our body is just ill-equipped to handle the daily, low-level stress: the morning commute, a bad boss, strained financial resources, troubles with school, and our poor diets.

Stressful Diets

Hays says that the number one thing that raises cortisol is a meal. "Every time you eat, a certain amount of food gets across into the blood and into the immune system. It's a way for your body to sample the environment." Then vitamin D and cortisol come out to turn down the immune response to that food. If the food we eat is particularly inflammatory, then cortisol levels will go up.

Hays describes the immune system as a "little herd of ponies." If the diet is full of anti-nutrients or inflammatory foods, then the ponies get out and run amok. If that goes on too long, then the cowboys, vitamin D and cortisol, need to come in and round them up. This is fine and continues to work as long as the cowboys are really good, but if you are using all your cortisol keeping the ponies in control, your body is left without its cowboys, which you need if you get a rash or the flu or your partner dies. Cortisol is your body's mechanism for dealing with inflammation. If the doctor starts prescribing you cortisol creams or steroids, says Hays, "you know your adrenal bank account is empty" and the result is very high-interest debt. "If you deal with stress by putting more cortisol in, you will produce diabetes." Instead, Hays encourages people to remove the stressor and rebuild the adrenal bank account, which can rebalance the system over time.

Improve Your Adrenal Bank Account

It is possible to invest back into the adrenal bank account so that the body has all of its resources available — including cortisol — when it needs them. Just like at the real bank, this means depositing more than you withdraw. "The main way to deposit is to sleep. If you aren't getting eight hours of sleep, you aren't making adequate deposits into your adrenal bank account."

The second part of the equation is to reduce the withdrawals. Food is the biggest source of withdrawals, so better food is key. For some people, especially those with thyroid problems, that may mean giving up particularly inflammatory foods such as gluten, as Hays has done. Other ways to reduce withdrawals from the adrenal bank account include meditation, better ways to deal with anger, and changing relationships and work place. "I have some people that are so high adrenaline that they set their alarms for every hour and then for five minutes they do nothing but breathe. If your adrenaline goes up and up and up all day you will get in bed at night and not be able to sleep."

Other important factors for adrenal balance include having sufficient vitamin D, which we are designed to get from the sun and store in fat cells and slowly release through the winter. In most places, people don't get enough vitamin D anymore and need supplementation. It is also important to reduce exposure to those environmental chemicals that can confuse the immune system.

Genetics are also a player, and some people are just born with higher adrenaline levels and have to work harder to keep adrenaline down. "Culturally we love these adrenaline junkies until they crash and burn," says Hays, who also says you can tell if you are one of these people because you will lose weight when under stress.

"Pregnancy is a motivator," reminds Hays. "Women will do things for a pregnancy or for a baby that they won't do for themselves." She also reminds us that when women change, they take the entire family with them. "Men and children all benefit from the changes women make in the home from [better] food to [eliminating] toxins."

Natural Help for Postpartum Depression and the "Baby Blues"

A period of hormonal fluctuation and increased stress is common after having a baby. One author described being pregnant as a time with the "stress-response brakes on." As the break comes off after birth, it can leave many women feeling overwhelmed and irritated. I remember the intense emotions of this time: the extreme pleasures and the challenges. I felt exhausted, I was often alone, and all of a sudden little things could become very big worries. Perhaps this is why I yelled at my mother and then burst into tears all because she wanted to bake the pizza without baking the crust first. (Sheesh. Sorry, Mom!)

One in ten women will experience more than just the usual amounts of sleeplessness, anxiety, and moodiness and will develop full-blown postpartum depression (PPD), characterized by severe mood swings, difficulty bonding with the baby, overwhelming fatigue, severe anxiety, and thoughts of harming yourself or your baby. Once a woman has had PPD, she has a 70 percent chance of having it again after subsequent pregnancies. If a woman is depressed before or during the pregnancy, or is dealing with other life stressors at the same time, she is at even greater risk.

The Causes of Postpartum Depression

The causes of PPD are at least threefold: hormonal, psychological, and neurochemical. When things are going really wrong in any one of these areas (say, hormones), or sort of wrong in a couple of areas (say psychological and neurological), this can lead to postpartum depression. To really cure a woman's PPD, she is likely to need support in all three areas.

Underlying the balance of all of these systems is nutrition, which feeds and balances the hormonal system, brain, and nervous system, as well as the body. Dr. Bethany Hays puts it simply: "You have just gone through nine months, plus breastfeeding, of having all your nutrients sucked away." She reminds women that the "body will feed the baby first," and that times of major hormonal fluctuation, such as the time before menstruation, menopause, early pregnancy, and postpartum, are difficult for women's brains, in part because of the stress that is put on the adrenals to try to balance out the huge fluctuations in estrogen and progesterone.

Treatment

PPD can be a severe, even life-threatening disease that should be taken seriously. Unfortunately, its treatment is often more symptomatic than healing. Serotonin-specific reuptake inhibitors (SSRIs), also referred to as anti-depressants, including sertraline, citalopram, escitalopram, paroxetine, and fluoxetine, are the most commonly prescribed drugs to treat PPD. They seem to work by pulling serotonin out of the brain cells and feeding it into the synapses, effectively speeding up the rate at which serotonin is used up by the brain. But therein lies the problem: speeding up the rate of use doesn't fix the underlying lack of serotonin. Those who decide to take the medication then are faced with the choice of either not breastfeeding to limit the baby's exposure, or exposing the baby to small amounts of the medication, which is transferred through the breast milk and reaches the baby's brain. Side effects can include a baby with a greater chance of developing colic and, for the mother, a greater risk of violence towards one's self and toward one's baby, and neurological symptoms that can continue beyond use, such as facial and body tics.

The Happiness Hormones

Serotonin is one of the "happiness hormones," a group that includes other hormones and neurochemicals that affect our mood and anxiety level. Serotonin doesn't work alone, and scientists don't fully understand its role in mood disorders, but they do know that it works closely with other happiness hormones, such as dopamine, to affect mood.

There are a couple of reasons why many women have low serotonin levels. The first one is nutritional. Many people simply don't have enough nutrients to create serotonin in the brain. The second reason is stress, or specific stressors, that interfere with the ability to use the nutritional precursors a person does have to make or use serotonin. In other words, stress increases our demand for serotonin and reduces our supply.

Remember, stress isn't just about bad thoughts. Stress can be caused by a bad day at work, and it can also be caused by chemicals in the environment, food sensitivities, and not getting enough sleep.

How Does Serotonin Work?

Within the nervous system, serotonin works together with other neurotransmitters — adrenaline, noradrenalin, and dopamine — to create a balance. When stress levels go up, the catecholamine side (with its stress-triggered hormones of adrenaline and noradrenalin) increase. When they increase, serotonin must increase, too, just to keep that scale balanced! It just so happens that many people's brains can't keep up with this increased demand.

The brain needs the essential amino acid tryptophan to make serotonin. An essential amino acid is one that the body can't make itself but needs to get from food or supplementation. Tryptophan works with other nutrients, such as iron, various B vitamins, and magnesium, to eventually become serotonin in the brain.

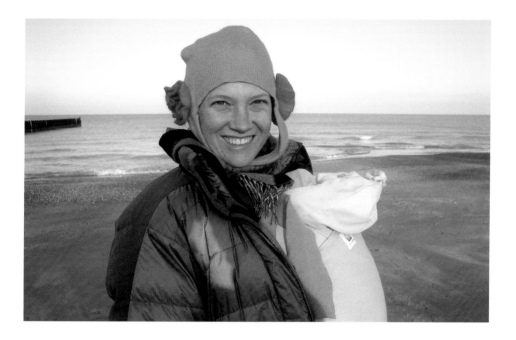

Eggs, beans, some seafood, red meat, chicken, turkey, and cheese all contain tryptophan. Unfortunately, most of the tryptophan that is ingested never makes it out of the intestinal tract, where it is used to help digest proteins. Serotonin also aids in digestion, but serotonin never makes it to the brain because it cannot cross the blood-brain barrier.

While a person can't eat serotonin, it is possible to take supplementation. Tryptophan and 5-hydroxy-tryptophan (5 HTP) can both cross the blood-brain barrier. Like tryptophan, 5 HTP is an amino acid and can become serotonin in the brain. Getting things across the blood-brain barrier can be tricky. It requires the help of a "ferrier protein" that works just like an actual ferry to get the amino acid and haul it across. There are a lot of other amino acids in that ferry lineup, however, and the tryptophan queue is longer, with more competing cars than the 5 HTP queue. (Living on an island, I know exactly how those poor, waiting amino acids feel.)

The Good News

Research suggests that nutritional supplementation, including things as simple as DHA (omega-3 fatty acids), can help relieve some postpartum depression symptoms. Other natural remedies for increasing serotonin include sunlight, gentle exercise, relaxation, mindfulness, massage, meditation, and sleep. There are also supplements that might help including 5 HTP, which is generally considered safe, although it is not usually advised in pregnant women. Gentler supplementations that can help during and after pregnancy include DHA, B vitamins, and magnesium. Read on for more tips.

Simplicity Parenting Is Parenting Simplified

Kim John Payne is the author of the Simplicity Parenting series of books and www.simplicityparenting.com. Payne started as a psychologist and while still in college worked and lived in a group home for gang-rescued and violent youth. While living there and studying, he became aware of the similarities between the youth around him and the emerging field of post-traumatic stress disorder (PTSD). The research, he says, was discussing combat veterans, but as he looked down the list of symptoms, he said he was "seeing it in my kids." These symptoms included controlling behaviours, overactive fight-or-flight response, difficulty with new things, and obsessive patterns of behaviour. There were even things such as not dressing appropriately for the environment — when it was cold, they would wear just a T-shirt — which he saw routinely playing out in these kids. "The hypothalamus controls temperature; this gets over-ridden by the primitive brain." It even went so far as sufferers having an "inability to properly taste food." These kids, like the veterans, needed high stimulation or they would cause conflict in their environment. Later he worked with young refugees from war zones, and again he saw similar behaviours.

Fast forward several years. "Imagine my surprise when I moved to the West and the kids coming through my door looked like the kids from my group home and from war-torn zones." They didn't dress appropriately, and they needed lots of flavouring in their foods — these were very stressed kids. But "there was nothing 'post' about it in these kids, it was ongoing; the highly stressed, fast-paced, too much, too sexy, too young, has become the new normal. It forces kids into a stressed zone. These kids aren't enjoying each other. They are surviving."

His book, *Simplicity Parenting*, "gives a voice to this feeling 'that something is wrong,'" he says. "Parents all around the world are feeling [it]: Everyone from Thunder Bay to Toronto to Vancouver to New York City to remote places I have travelled in Africa, people saying there is something wrong." He adds, "All kids are quirky. If we add accumulative stress to that, that quirk becomes problematic and may even become a disorder."

But there is a silver lining; Payne has trained a veritable army of Simplicity Parenting coaches and parent educators, and they all say that "while on one hand the irritated quirk can be a disorder, the soothed quirk becomes a gift."

"Given rhythm, safety, a life that doesn't overwhelm them, no screens or low screens, a lot of downtime, a lot of nature, the gift of the ADHD child is that they are incredibly motivated and motivate others." He adds that when the child's fight-or-flight tendency calms down, they can "do things in the right time, in the right place, and at the right volume."

"Simplifying isn't about going back into the past, it's about a child being able to show their gifts to the world." Simplicity Parenting coaches have the benefit of learning from what has worked with thousands of families. They help families realize their children's gifts by simplifying the environment, simplifying and strengthening rhythm, simplifying schedules, and filtering out overwhelming information. These four principles apply to pregnancy, too; in fact, says Payne, they are "potentized in pregnancy. When you are pregnant you see the world peeled back: you start to see what is needed and what is not, where you begin to ask the good questions, you have the care of this being inside you."

1. **Around the house.** Simplify. Get rid of stuff. Declutter. Ask your friends to come for a day and help. And, Payne cautions, be "careful about things like baby showers." If you do one, "ask your friends to come together to get one thing: like a really good stroller that will be there for your sixth child." Just one thing! For instance, one thing from the mother's side and one from the spouse or partner's side. (I'd recommend an organic mattress and a great, real wood crib, co-sleeper, or bed.) "Nesting is sorting out the essential from the nonessential."
2. **Establish healthy rhythms** around mealtimes, bedtime, and exercise. Rhythms are gentle and soothing and calm the parasympathetic nervous system. "A child's nervous system directly feeds off ours. The formation of a child's brain directly feeds off of ours. Babies thrive on rhythm." If you don't have rhythm and the baby arrives, it's a lot to deal with, trying to lay a new rhythm while learning all about a new life. Payne says that "even in utero the baby starts tuning in to the mother's rhythm, and when it arrives it will already be tuned in."
3. **Dial back on scheduling commitments.** A mother's nervous system will benefit from doing less and having fewer commitments; she will feel healthier and be more rested, says Payne. Many women hit a wall after a baby comes and they realize how much less they can get done in a day. "To anticipate that and start dialling back on scheduling means that by the time the baby arrives you have lessened your need for adrenaline and cortisol and your own need for activity, and it's more likely you will be happy being home with baby and enjoying the little things, because your own system will have attuned."
4. **Filter out overwhelming information.** "Avoid listening to the news or cut back to once a day; cut back on your screen time — computers, gaming; filter out a lot of the 'horribles,'" says Payne. If this seems unnecessary or impossible, he adds, "there is time to emerge back into the world, but during pregnancy is one of the few times that we have a really good reason for focusing on something other than the terrible violence of the world. To surround one's self with goodness and hope."

"If you understand the power of less, by the time the baby arrives, you are ready and you're adjusted." Payne says these four practices above are especially beneficial for fathers, adoptive parents, and women wanting to ward off postpartum depression. "If one follows the four principles of simplicity, you don't have to do anything, you just have to do less." Less is a practice that helps many parents deal with the mounting stressors of modern-day living.

How to Green the Fourth Trimester and Prepare for Postpartum Bliss

Here are a series of action steps listed from ♥♥♥ (biggest impact, and possibly more work) to ♥ (quick and easy) to help you ease into and be happier in the postpartum period.

1. ♥♥♥ **Eat for the postpartum brain during pregnancy.** Dr. Bethany Hays recommends focusing on omega-3 fatty acids (think fish oils), proper amino acids (which are used to make those "happiness hormones" and brain chemicals and help digest and break down proteins), and B vitamins (which help with methylation — the formation and breakdown of just about every brain chemical) while pregnant. It's not too late, however, to benefit from them whenever you start.

2. ♥♥♥ **Sleep.** Hays says this is particularly important for "high-adrenaline" women, whose cortisol levels will rise if they don't get enough sleep, if they experience the stress associated with caring for a new baby, or if they have an underlying genetic predisposition. As cortisol levels go up, so will anxiety, and this can also result in depression. These women need to get their adrenaline down. The first thing they need is adequate sleep, says Hays. At the first sign of trouble, ideally before, get help! She recommends arranging for three nights off to sleep. (She isn't saying not to breastfeed. She recommends having somebody you can pass the baby to directly after feeding, or to pump so you can sleep.) That old adage, "sleep when the baby sleeps," can truly help!

3. ♥♥♥ **Breastfeed.** Research suggests that breastfeeding can help stave off postpartum depression. It can be even more effective if the woman is making sure to get enough brain nutrients and other nutritional support. "Eat when the baby eats," says Hays.

4. ♥♥ **Assess your stress.** If you are so exhausted you can't imagine ever pulling yourself out of your deep, dark hole and you have trouble eliciting positive thoughts, you might be suffering from adrenal fatigue, hyperthyroidism, or postpartum depression. Sleep and great nutrition can help with these things, but you may also need the advice of a doctor or other healthcare practitioner.

5. ♥♥ **Develop a nourishing family rhythm.** Many of the birth providers and parenting gurus interviewed for this book reflected that women with

simplified daily routines — with fewer commitments, obligations, and visitors — were more likely to have smoother and happier postpartum periods. Give yourself time to get to know the baby and develop a daily rhythm that nourishes, rather than rushes, the entire family. Read the **Simplicity Parenting** section on pages 186–87 to learn how.

6. ♥♥ **Try supportive natural therapies** such as herbs, essential oils, yoga, and meditation.

7. ♥ **Bio-identical progesterone supplementation** might help some women with postpartum depression. "It's not my first solution to PPD," says Hays, "but it can be effective and relatively harmless…." Progesterone, however, won't work with high-adrenaline women, because in these women the progesterone will just be made into more cortisol. "These women just get more irritable, sleepless, and depressed when put on progesterone," warns Hays. Women who it does benefit may feel calmer, lose weight, and sleep better.

The Day After: What to Have on Hand for the Days Immediately After Baby Arrives

1. ♥♥♥ **A plan so you can stay in bed** as much as possible. Ideally, stay close to home for six weeks after birth. Your baby, breast milk supply, and own healing will all benefit from doing less. Even adoptive parents and partners benefit from doing less during this period. Midwife Kate Koyote recommends that parents during this time turn off their cellphones and stay off social media. "One of the basic rules: Sleep when your baby is sleeping. You might be awake all night long. The computer and social media is one of the things that keep a brain going. The social interaction is having visitors — who bring meals — it's not social media."

2. ♥♥♥ **A plan for getting nutrition-rich, organic, whole foods.** If you are nursing, you need more calories than pregnant moms: about 800 more calories a day. Look into help getting nourishing meals, even if you are an adoptive parent or a partner. A postpartum doula can come and help you nurse, take the baby while you sleep, or help prepare a meal. There are also services available today that will deliver ready-to-prepare meals: a recipe, all the food you need, and everything pre-measured and chopped. Other services will deliver fresh, organic food right to your door. Save yourself the shopping, and prepare early to help you get the food you need.

3. ♥♥♥ **Many, many nutritious frozen meals.** "A meal, please" is the answer for everyone who asks "What can I get you?" or "Where are you registered?" After the birth, ask everybody who wants to visit to bring a meal, and ask them to wait to come for at least a week, maybe more, after the birth.

4. ♥♥♥ **A plan for breastfeeding support.** Assess who you will call for regular support and more specialized support — perhaps an experienced friend who you've asked in advance and the number of a lactation consultant, just in case. Have a breastfeeding book on hand. Just about any book, even used and outdated, will have loads of practical advice that can really save the day (or night) when things aren't going well at 2:00 a.m. (See the **Further Reading** section for some of my favourite books.) As well, if you can afford it, get a hand pump; you will use it even if you don't plan to regularly pump. It can be a saviour for assessing or increasing supply, helping with clogged ducts, or just pumping for a night's rest. If you know you won't or can't breastfeed, arrange to have some breast milk or homemade formula on hand.

5. ♥♥♥ **A postpartum doula** or a relative or close friend who will come during the first six weeks to do laundry, fold, sweep, and cook. Consider having somebody come at night so that you can get three nights of solid sleep, or sleep with just one nursing.

6. ♥♥♥ **A plan for getting support.** If you have had anxiety or depression before the birth, you are at greater risk for postpartum depression. Have a proactive plan for getting additional nutritional support and counselling, and surround yourself with fewer crazy relatives and more truly helpful partners. Peer support such as can be found in a breastfeeding group, a mother's group, or a play group can be extremely helpful for all mothers, especially those at risk for postpartum depression. Online support can also be great, but being online can also have a negative impact on people's moods and disrupt their sleep and their early bonding time. As well, it doesn't have the same neurological benefits as meeting in person with other new mothers.

7. ♥♥♥ **A safe place for the baby to sleep.** Have a safe place for the baby without pillows or duvets. Ideally, this would include a truly natural, toxin-free mattress.

8. ♥♥ **Will you encapsulate the placenta?** If so, you must have it all planned out beforehand.

9. ♥♥ **A green diaper option.** Have a diaper option ready — the simpler the better for the first three months because you will use *a lot*. You will do a lot of laundry during this time anyway, so simple, pre-fold cotton diapers or a cloth diaper service are perfect. Or get unbleached, unscented disposable diapers or compostable ones. Wait to make your final diaper choice until after the baby grows a bit; three months is ideal.

10. ♥♥ **Understand blood flow after birth.** It can be a lot more than women realize. Talk with your healthcare provider and plan for it by getting enough pads. I recommend reusable cotton menstrual pads. Or you may want disposable pads; just make sure they are unbleached, organic, and without fragrance, because you want only the gentlest, healthiest products close to your body. Read up on home remedies, such as making your own frozen witch hazel compresses. Another trick is to fill a condom with water and freeze it and wrap it in cotton. Place this against the perineum.

11. ♥♥ **Natural remedies to support your postpartum nourishment.** These include herbal teas, essential oils, and homeopathic remedies to support the mother's healing and nourishment, breast milk supply, and relaxation See **The Natural Postpartum Handbook** at the end of this chapter for ideas.

12. ♥ **Organic cotton swaddling blankets.** Babies love to be swaddled, and even if you never swaddle the baby, you will use those little cotton blankets

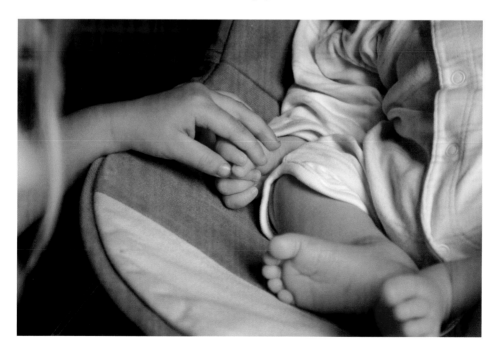

to put the baby to rest on the floor or on your bed, to cover the new car seat, or to protect your shirt from the milk and spit-up flowing everywhere.

13. ♥ **Truly natural baby toiletries.** A baby needs very, very little in the first few weeks. They won't be running around getting dirty yet, so no soaps or shampoos are needed. You can use edible oils for moisturizing or you can buy a few things beforehand to have at the ready. Just make sure all the ingredients are organic and edible, because the baby's skin is extremely porous and can absorb most everything readily. My family doctor recommended just washing the baby in the sink when changing the dirty diaper, so with my second, the baby changing area was on the counter next to the sink and involved almost no effort. Where will you change your baby?

14. ♥ **Do you still have that birth ball?** A yoga ball is great as an alternative to a chair for the prenatal period, can be quite nice during labour, and after labour it's a great tool for the partner to use as an alternative to "rocking" the baby. In my experience, babies love bouncing second only to breastfeeding, and my ball bought me many hours of extra sleep as my husband bounced our baby through the night.

15. ♥ **A natural rubber pacifier** once the breastfeeding relationship is safely established can be a real blessing. Not all babies have a strong sucking reflex, but for those who do, nothing helps like a pacifier. Beware that the plastic ones at the drug store can release endocrine-mimicking plasticizers.

16. ♥ **A peri bottle.** That's a handheld squirt bottle, usually plastic, that you fill with warm water to rinse your vagina for as long as you are sore after the birth.

What to Have on Hand for Three Months After Birth

1. ♥♥♥ **Healthy snacks and meals** to support your continued nourishment. It can take three years for a mother, even one doing everything "right," to recover from pregnancy and birth. Remember, your blood and brain and tissue are all made up from the nutrients you take in, and while you are nursing you are still passing on much of what you take in and have stored to your baby.

2. ♥♥♥ **The number of a pelvic floor physical therapist,** or learn exercises to do at home. This is more than Kegels; my pelvic floor physical therapist

said that most women actually need to learn to relax as well as strengthen, and often Kegels just cause a woman to hold tension in her nether parts.

3. ♥♥ **Cloth diapers.** There are services that will let you try out different kinds of diapers before buying. There are also diaper cleaning services, where you just rent the diapers and somebody else picks them up and washes them.

4. ♥ **A sleep sack.** Sometime between three months and six months, your baby will bust out of her swaddle no matter how much duct tape you use. (Okay, don't really use duct tape; it's not a very green option for sleeping.) An organic cotton sleep sack — sometimes they come with Velcro straps to help hold those flailing arms at bay — is a safe alternative to blankets for a baby and are almost as effective as the swaddle for helping with sleep.

5. ♥ **A lovey.** This is a little ragdoll-type thing, often made of terry cotton, that is organic and natural and that the baby can chew on or cuddle with. You can wear it close to your body to give it your own smell.

6. ♥ **Natural teething supplies.** Oh yes, it can start so much earlier than I ever realized. Have an amber teething necklace, a wooden rattle, and a few natural remedies on hand for when your baby suddenly starts drooling and howling with this new sensation.

The Natural Postpartum Handbook

· ·

I have found home remedies are a great way to feel more empowered as a mama. I am known among my friends as the person who will pull out a tub of herbal cream or a homeopathic tincture and say "try this." Remember, however, that these are home remedies meant as a guide to empower your healing path, not a substitute for medical advice. A family doctor or naturopathic physician will be your trusted partner for many years to come. If you don't already have one, the earlier you find someone, the easier it will be to trust them when you have a true medical need. I found a great family physician in Chicago after my first baby and specifically looked for someone with experience with breastfed and home-birthed babies. I was so appreciative of his patient guidance and support that I withstood a two-year waiting list to get the family doctor I wanted after I moved to Canada. I have never regretted the wait.

Herbs for the Baby Blues

My friend calls lemon balm leaves a "mother's little helper," and that is especially true during the postpartum period when one or two cups a day of tea made from lemon balm leaves for a couple weeks will do wonders for depression, melancholy, and hysteria, according to *Wise Woman Herbal for the Childbearing Year* by Susun Weed. For more severe depression, a tincture made of blessed (or milk) thistle, likely available at your local health food store or natural apothecary, can help (or drink two cups a day of milk thistle tea). Read the nutritional suggestions in this chapter for additional ideas for helping the typical baby blues, and if things don't get better or you feel that you might harm yourself or your baby, immediately seek medical help.

Susun Weed's Wise Woman Herbal Postpartum Depression Brew

Ingredients:
14g dried, shredded licorice root
28g dried, crushed raspberry leaf
28g dried, finely cut rosemary leaves
28g dried, cut skullcap

Directions:
Combine ingredients and use 2 teaspoons (10g) per cup of boiling water.

Perineum Care

You can use herbs on your perineum as well. Matraea, the midwifery group started by Kate Koyote, makes organic teas for pregnancy and postpartum care. Their perineal wash is very popular. It includes comfrey root, comfrey leaf, chickweed, plantain leaf, calendula flowers, lavender blossoms, and yarrow flowers. You can make your own by adding any or all of these herbs, and red raspberry leaf as well, to a bath. Add about one cup in a hot bath, to which you can also add 1/4 cup of pure Epsom or sea salt. Or, you can brew the herbal mixture, cool, and add to water in a peri bottle for direct application, or add it to your cotton menstrual pads and freeze for a perineum Popsicle. If you heavily dilute the mixture, you can add a bit to the area around the baby's umbilical cord to help with healing.

Essential oils can also be used for the perineum. Try 10 drops lavender and 10 drops frankincense with 1 tablespoon (15ml) of water in a spray or peri bottle.

Mastitis Relief

Getting a breast infection is like being run over by a train, and your boob hurts. When I had my one breast infection in six years of nursing, my breast hardly hurt, but I felt like I had just run a long, hard cross-country race. If your breast becomes engorged or you develop a full case of mastitis (an infection of the breast tissue that results in breast pain, swelling, warmth, and redness, often accompanied by fever and chills), there are home remedies that may help, but don't wait! A full-fledged breast infection can become quite serious and may need medical attention if it persists.

Nurse and Drain

Mastitis usually starts with a plugged milk duct. The longer you breastfeed, the easier it becomes to tell when this is starting to happen. I had a duct on my left breast on the side near where an underwire might press that would drain slower than the rest. When I got mastitis, it was from this duct getting clogged. Keep nursing through a clogged duct and drain the breast every time, including those reluctant ducts. Use some vegetable oil to massage those sluggish ducts, pressing toward the nipple. Warm showers also help: if a clogged duct gets really bad, stand in the shower with the hot stream of water hitting the difficult area and massage and express the breast in the shower, or use the warm water to prepare the breast for nursing. Try to start feeding on the difficult breast. You can also try to position the baby so that the chin (or nose, if that's impossible) is pointed toward the clogged duct. This may direct the greatest sucking pressure on the clogged duct.

Cabbage Compresses

Green cabbage leaves reduce supply. That's great in major cases of engorgement or infection, but not great when you are trying to establish a new breastfeeding relationship, so use with care. Take apart the cabbage, leaving full, clean leaves. You can chill if you like. I removed the biggest part of the stem. Wrap the leaves around the breast, but avoid the nipple itself. Leave on the engorged breast for 20 minutes, or until they get warm and start to wither.

Natural Flu Remedies

Sometimes, a woman will start feeling flu-like before she even realizes she has an infection. Some doctors say that if a breastfeeding mom thinks she has the flu, it's likely a breast infection (or the one leads to the other). Raw garlic and echinacea herbs can be safe and effective for preventing infections and helping stimulate the immune system naturally. Combined with sleep and the remedies above, you can quickly stop mastitis from becoming a full infection.

Nipple Relief

Cracked or bleeding nipples can be a sign that the latch isn't quite right. For the first few days, well, it can just be a lot to get used to. But once breastfeeding is established, nursing shouldn't hurt. If it does, it can be tweaked so that it doesn't. After fixing, or along with fixing, the latch, you can help your nipples to heal. With cracked nipples, feed on the cracked side second because the baby will often nurse more gently on the second side.

Applying breast milk to the sore nipple is entirely safe and has been shown to be effective both because it is naturally antibacterial and because it is warm and moisturizing (both of which can help). Try a natural lanolin cream to help maintain the internal moisture of the skin. Essential oils may also provide relief. Try applying one drop of lavender or Roman chamomile on the nipple after feeding so that it will be gone before the next feeding.

Breast Milk Supply

Remember, it is very rare that a woman can't produce enough milk, yet supply is nevertheless an issue that women frequently face. In short, that means that in almost all cases, a lack of supply can be fixed with help. This can come from a doctor who specializes in breastfeeding, a lactation consultant, or even a really knowledgeable friend. Options range from correcting the latch or drinking herbal teas to using a supplementer — a contraption that works like a bottle and connects to the breast itself — or taking a prescription medicine (see more in the **Breastfeeding Breakdown** on page 161). Remember, breastfeeding works on supply and demand, so the more "demand" from breastfeeding frequency, pumping, and thoroughly draining each breast, the more milk that should be created.

Eating plenty of highly nutritious food, drinking ample clean water, and getting adequate sleep will help your body produce what is demanded. Certain herbs can help with this, but others can hinder. Helpful herbs include alfalfa leaf, which can both help with milk supply and vitamin K levels, as well as blessed thistle, comfrey leaves, fennel, fenugreek (and other strong-tasting seeds), goat's rue, nettle, and milk thistle. Foods rich in carotene (usually richer and better-absorbed cooked) can also help, including all kind of cooked greens, apricots, asparagus, green beans, carrots, tomato sauces, and peas. Eat these foods with lots of fat for better absorption.

Another *Wise Woman* cure includes barley water — just cook barley with extra water and drink the broth that's made. You can add a teaspoon of fennel seeds, too.

Essential oils for milk supply support can include one drop of basil added to one drop liquid coconut oil or other edible oil. Dab it on the body, avoiding the nipples.

Herbs that may hinder production include lots of either peppermint or spearmint and sage. As well, birth control pills, decongestants, and even supplemental melatonin can decrease milk supply. There are a number of herbs that can also be harmful to mother and baby (see the list on page 95 in **The Natural Pregnancy Handbook**); however, the amounts found in a meal shouldn't be a problem. Make sure your healthcare provider knows you're breastfeeding, or get familiar with the list if making your own herbal remedies.

Mother's Milk Infusion

There are a number of ready-made, organic herbal teas on the market to help with milk supply. These include Matraea's Rumina's Milk Tea, Traditional Medicine's Mother's Milk, and Earth Mama Angel Baby's Milkmaid Tea. You can also make your own. Susun Weed, the famous herbalist mentioned earlier in this chapter, particularly recommends taking breastfeeding supportive herbs as an infusion. Remember to always use organic herbs. The basic recipe is to take 28 grams of herbs (placing them in a large canning jar works well) and pour over it a litre of boiling water. Put the lid on and let it steep for four hours to overnight. Strain. You can drink it hot, cold, or at room temperature. The leftovers can be refrigerated for up to 48 hours.

Susun Weed's Triple Blessing Brew

Make an infusion as above using 14g of dried blessed thistle and 14g of dried nettle. Before nursing, heat the infusion and pour it over 1 teaspoon (5ml) of anise, cumin, fennel, caraway, or coriander and brew for five minutes. Drink. Nurse. Enjoy.

Natural Remedies for Jaundice

Jaundice is common in newborns, and it seems to be more common and lasts a bit longer in breastfed babies. The good news is that in most cases jaundice is harmless and can easily be treated at home. The bad news is that not all doctors are up to date on the current research on jaundice and may encourage practices such as taking a breastfeeding break and feeding the baby water, sugar water, or formula. These practices are no longer supported by the evidence.

Jaundice occurs because babies are born with more red blood cells than they need. When the liver breaks down these cells, it results in bilirubin, which is the cause of the yellow pigment that can show up in the skin and eyes of the newborn. The baby's liver, just like all of her organs of detoxification, is still forming and, thus, she isn't very efficient or fast at disposing of the bilirubin. Eventually the baby will process the bilirubin and poop it out.

This normal, physiological jaundice might take a week or two or even three to diminish. Breastfed babies tend to have bilirubin levels on average of 14.8 milligrams, versus 12.4 milligrams in the formula-fed baby, and there doesn't seem to be any harm in this at all. According to Dr. William Sears, pediatrician and author of *The Baby Book*, it isn't usually necessary to treat normal jaundice when bilirubin levels are less than 20 milligrams. The best ways to prevent levels rising are in line with getting baby off to a great breastfeeding start, and this includes lots and lots of breastfeeding, which also helps with the baby's poop, which is how he eliminates the bilirubin. Jaundiced babies can be sleepier, so you may need to wake the baby to encourage him to nurse.

My grandma always told stories of leaving the babies in her college home ec course in the sunlight. This, indeed, can help. If, however, that's not an option, try a full spectrum light bulb for you both at home. If the baby's levels rise to 20 milligrams or above, the doctor will likely want him to undergo phototherapy treatment. The good news is that there are now options for this, such as photo-optic blankets, that can be used at home so the mother-and-baby breastfeeding relationship isn't disturbed. Sometimes jaundice can occur, as it did with my sister, after a particularly busy day (for her it was a week postpartum). She was running her older children around to sporting events, taking the baby for a postpartum check-up, and feeling all the stresses of new motherhood. In her case, the best treatment was taking a few days totally off to rest in a sunny bedroom and breastfeed. The mother will benefit from rest and drinking lots of water. If you're still worried about normal jaundice, some mamas take liver tonic herbs to pass on to the baby through the breast milk. These include a few drops each of burdock root, dandelion root, and yellow dock root.

Natural Remedies for Thrush

For a number of weeks after birth, the baby's immune system is suppressed. The theory in the microbiome world is that this serves the purpose of making it easier

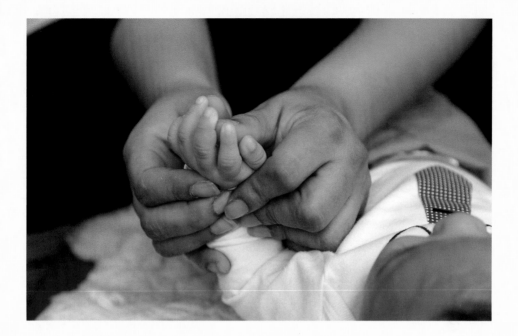

for the beneficial bacteria of the mother to colonize the baby. The baby is exposed to this beneficial bacteria beginning in the womb, while travelling through the birth canal, and afterward through breast milk.

Nevertheless, many babies will develop thrush, which is an overgrowth of yeast in the mouth, and they are especially vulnerable if the mother or baby has received antibiotics before, during, or directly after birth. It can look like cottage cheese or lots of milk residue on the tongue, inner cheeks, and roof of the mouth. Most cases of thrush will just go away on their own, but if it's causing your baby discomfort or you are passing it between your nipples and the baby, then you may want to try a home remedy. You may consider giving a small dose of probiotic to a newborn baby that has been exposed to antibiotics to prevent thrush, says Kelly Bonyata, IBCLC, on the breastfeeding support website www.kellymom.com. This can be done by having the breastfeeding mother take the probiotics, some of which will be passed to the baby along with the naturally occurring probiotics in the breast milk. It is possible to give small amounts of probiotic directly to a baby suffering from thrush if you have a super pure source of probiotic. This can be done by dipping your finger into the powder (open the capsule) and letting the baby suck it off your finger. I'd personally wait to do this until you've tried the breastfeeding route or if the baby is not being breastfed. Other home remedies include dissolving baking soda in warm, filtered water and rubbing the final mixture inside the baby's mouth. You can treat your grownup self for yeast overgrowth, as well, which will help keep you from exchanging the infection back and forth. Eat lots of plain, organic, whole milk yogourt, take your own probiotic supplements, and restrict your intake of all sugars and simple carbohydrates until it is cleared up.

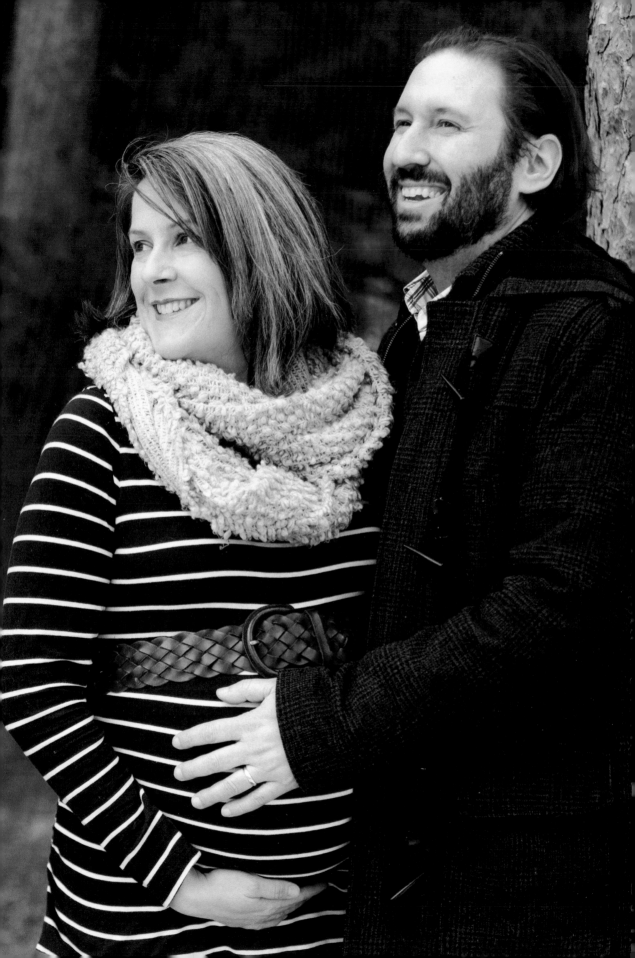

chapter eight

Greening for Your Future Fertility

· ·

I have met dozens of families who suffered from infertility; then, like a switch, it was no longer an issue. The switch for many of these families seemed to be their first child. A few of the couples I knew adopted, others had IVF or fertility drug support, and still others just waited a long time, yet somehow their second, third, and even fourth children happened as if by magic. I think now it is because we make so many healthy changes for the sake of our children, and these changes improve the health of our whole family. Indeed, they can improve the health of our entire world and our future.

Fertility isn't just a switch, however; it is a barometer of health, for women and for men. "To be fertile is to be in as balanced a state as a human can be," says Dr. Spence Pentland, the TCM doctor and fertility book author. There are few losses more dear to a person than not being able to conceive the family of their dreams.

"I promise, you will be a mother," a friend said to me while I floated in that space post-miscarriage and pre-child. I believed her. This friend's path to becoming a mother had been a ten-year journey with multiple pregnancy losses and just about every known fertility treatment. Her point: that our journeys to parenthood may not be what we expect, but that for those of us with resources in the developed world, we have many options. While many of us crave the experience of growing a child in our womb and birthing her ourselves, there are many other paths to creating a family. I grew up in a family where not one of the four siblings claims the same set of birth parents: I know that we love children just as much whether we bare them ourselves or not. However we become parents, the process links us forever to our children. This is never more evident than in how we care for our health: by doing so — mothers and fathers — we care for our children. We know more everyday about how to achieve and restore fertility both as a baseline of our own health and to fulfill our dreams of family.

The Research

Few women know that about 25 percent of all women have experienced a miscarriage. One-in-six pregnancies end this way, with the incidence increasing with the age of the mother. It helped me to talk about my miscarriage because I soon discovered I wasn't alone in this common experience. I also realized what the statistics verify: the majority of women who have miscarried eventually carry babies to term. Miscarriage is often caused by genetic defects — sometimes caused by environmental toxins — but rarely caused by something a woman *did*. In other words, it's not the mother-to-be's fault for eating the wrong food, exercising too much or too little, or having that glass of wine before she knew she had conceived. There are things, though, that women — and men — can do to help detoxify and prepare the body in preparation for the next pregnancy.

Infertility has nearly doubled in 20 years, effecting up to 16 percent of couples in Canada. It's estimated that about 11 percent of women are infertile. It's harder to estimate with men, but the research is clear that men's infertility is on the rise and about 1 percent of men have no sperm in their ejaculate.

Fertility Is Also About Men

In conversations about fertility, it is often women that become the focus. Yet, when I was researching this book, the fertility experts I spoke with said it's time to look more at the men.

Men are less fertile than they were a few decades age. The quality and amount of sperm is declining, and fast, while simultaneously there is a rise in male genital birth defects. In 2005, the largest study ever done on male fertility showed that counts fell by one-third in a 16-year period in over 26,600 French men. The study showed nearly a 2 percent annual decrease and took the average sperm count from 74 million per millilitre to about 50 million. The quality of sperm is also declining, so much so that the WHO has officially changed their definition of "normal" from greater than 60 percent healthy, un-deformed sperm in a man's ejaculate in 1980 to just 4 percent healthy, un-deformed sperm. This dramatic shift in "normal" occurred in less than 40 years. While there is ongoing debate as to how much quality sperm is really needed to create a pregnancy — after all, it just takes one lucky sperm to create an embryo — what is clear is that more sperm of good quality increase pregnancy rates, and 4 percent isn't much.

"Sperm is a great base line indicator of what is going on in the environment. Our sperm are sensitive to environmental toxins," says Pentland. Indeed, the most comprehensive study yet done on specific environmental toxins and their effects on couples getting pregnant suggest that the male's role is every bit as threatened as the woman's, and perhaps even more sensitive to current exposures.

The Longitudinal Investigation of Fertility and the Environment (LIFE) study followed 500 couples for 12 months as they attempted to conceive and measured their blood for the presence of 63 organic pollutants common in almost all North Americans and Europeans. The results suggested that greater exposures to certain environmental toxins did indeed affect the time to pregnancy. In women, the greatest associations were to persistent organic pollutants (POPs), including PCBs and perflourinated compounds. In men, the greatest associations, up to 29 percent reduction in his partner achieving pregnancy, were with an ever greater number of POPs, including seven different PCBs and one pesticide (DDE). These effects were so strong that in some cases they reduced fertility as much as age.

That's not all. Low-quality sperm may increase the incidence of miscarriage, and, in viable pregnancies, sperm quality may be linked to conditions such as metabolic syndrome, diabetes, osteoporosis, and testicular and prostate cancer.

There is good news. These same studies suggest that male fertility responds to the same health practices as female fertility: practising proper nutrition, maintaining healthy weight, avoiding excessive alcohol consumption, limiting caffeine consumption, and using acupuncture and certain Chinese herbs. The nature of sperm also means that men may be able to improve their fertility faster and more dramatically than women. The long and short of it is that the health of the man is important in making babies, and good fertility practices for women are also vital for men.

The Fifth Vital Sign: Fertility Tracking as a Window to Health

The Justisse Method of fertility awareness is about more than preventing or achieving pregnancy, says Geraldine Matus, founder of Justisse Healthworks for Women and Justisse College. "It can be used as a window into a woman's endocrine system," the second most vital system after the central nervous system. "If the endocrine symptom isn't working, you aren't working." Because of this, she considers a woman's cycle the fifth vital sign, after blood pressure, body temperature, heart rate, and respiration rate.

"As soon as our reproductive health declines, our whole life health declines." She compares the stresses that women face today to the straw that broke the camel's back. "Wi-Fi, stress, dietary pollution, what are the stressors on the camel's back that breaks a person? One person will say it is high fructose corn syrup and another lead in water." Ultimately, "it's epigenetics: the environment determines how the genetic information is realized."

A Healthy Cycle Is About 28 to 35 Days

- Day one of the cycle begins with a true, healthy menstrual bleed, which is a bright red bleed that last three to five days and is neither too heavy nor light in that time, nor should it be extremely painful.

- This is followed by a period of follicle and egg development, in which there will be no cervical fluid. The length of this period is variable, depending on the woman's health and environmental factors.
- The last day of that type of mucus is associated with an ovulatory event when the ovum is released to the fallopian tube.
- This is followed by a 12- to 14-day secretory phase when the uterus lining prepares for the possibility of conception and the mucus discharge dries, the basal body temperature rises, and the cervical os closes.

Cycles that include extreme pain, premenstrual syndrome, and extreme moodiness are signs that something is wrong with the system. It is possible to "see" what is happening with a woman's endocrine system by tracking these three biomarkers: cervical fluid, basal body temperature, and position of the cervix, all of which only take a few minutes a day to observe and record.

A healthy woman with a healthy cycle can use the knowledge of her cycle to help achieve pregnancy. Conception is possible only on ovulation day, and a woman is only fertile the few days every cycle that she has cervical mucus. Preventing pregnancy naturally by charting her three biomarkers and practising abstinence during the windows when she is able to receive has been proven to be effective: up to 99.4 percent when followed perfectly. This is not the same as the rhythm method, which isn't as effective because it depends on mathematical calculations to predict fertile days, rather than actually tracking the body's indicators of fertility. You can learn more about fertility tracking and download an app to get started at www.justisse.ca.

If You Have Previously Used Hormonal Birth Control

If you have previously used hormonal birth control — and who hasn't these days — you will likely need help recovering your optimal health, ideally before your next pregnancy. Hormonal birth control can deplete the body of key nutrients, including thyroid hormones and zinc, which are both crucial for reproductive health. "There is evidence that the longer a woman is on hormonal contraception, the longer it may take for her cycle to return," says woman's health writer Jennifer Block. "So if you [want] to be pregnant, think a year or two ahead," she says, as it can take that long to be ovulating regularly. She cautions that many women have been on the pill since they were young to treat conditions such as irregular periods, endometriosis, and polycystic ovarian syndrome. "These women often then go off the pill and the symptoms return with a vengeance because the reality is that the pill hasn't been treating the symptoms but masking them."

"It's a myth, this idea that hormonal birth control is harmless," says midwife Geraldine Matus. She has seen hundreds of women struggle to rebuild their fertility after using hormonal birth control. "Being on the pill is not like being pregnant." Hormonally, it is more like being perimenopausal or menopausal, a state that ages a woman quickly. It can take a few years of a woman tracking her fertility and working with a helper to recover fertility, but it is possible, says Matus. She recommends learning to track your fertility as a start.

"One of the deficiencies of modern gynecology is that we aren't effectively treating these conditions, we are just masking them with pharmaceutical hormones," says Block. She cautions that many of these same women are later diagnosed with infertility and end up taking more synthetic hormones in order to get pregnant, and "we still aren't treating their underlying health." The answer is to plan well in advance to help restore your body to health.

Child Spacing

While many parents these days think of child spacing in terms of getting time off work or affording a large enough home, those wise in traditional ways say that child spacing is better determined by the health of the mother. The Weston A. Price Foundation, based on the work of dentist and anthropological researcher Dr. Weston Price, recommends at least three years as the minimal amount of time

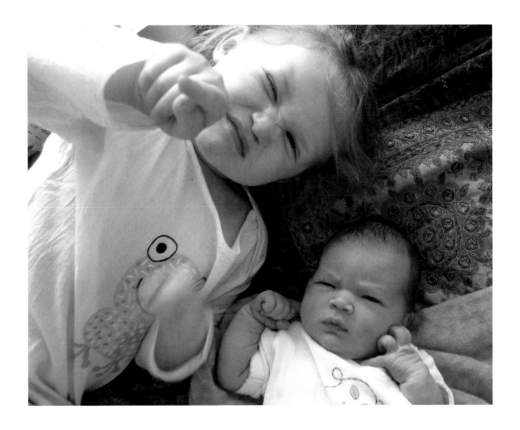

Ten Steps to Overcoming Infertility

Dr. Spence Pentland is the author of *Being Fertile* and a doctor of Traditional Chinese Medicine (TCM), which is a degree akin to a medical doctor (MD) that usually involves about five years of post-graduate training, hundreds of hours of clinical practice, and provincial (or state) licensure exams. TCM doctors use herbs, acupuncture, diet, and holistic examination tools to assess the state of the physical and energetic body and create a plan towards balance. He is a father of three, and this appreciation and love of family has guided him to help others achieve their dreams of family. "I love treating fertility more than any other condition," says Pentland, which is why he has made this his focus of for the past 15 years. He also conducts clinical research on IVF and acupuncture, and does research into the effects of environmental contaminants on fertility.

Pentland's first bit of advice toward overcoming infertility is to use TCM: "Your body's innate desire is to be balanced and healthy. Acupuncture gives it a helping hand." There is a growing body of research to back these claims. A 2016 study done by the British Homerton University Hospital found that using acupuncture on women trying to conceive by IVF doubled their chances of conceiving: 46.2 percent of the treatment group conceived versus only 21.7 of the women in the IVF only group. Acupuncture for the father, though presently unstudied, seems likely to have positive effects as well.

His other nine steps include many of the topics covered in this book, including setting holistic goals that recognize fertility as a sign of whole body health, learning to listen to what your body is telling you, nurturing your spirit, using diet and supplements for both the future mama and papa to achieve health, partaking in enjoyable levels of exercise, becoming aware of fertility-taxing toxins and how to avoid them, being open to trying other forms of holistic treatment, understanding the assisted reproductive technology options and integrating them as necessary into your holistic health path, and remembering that men's health and well-being is half the picture and that many of the same practices that will improve a woman's fertility will also help a man. Two cautions: look for TCM doctors who are licensed by your province or state (www.aborm.org is a great place to start looking); and use herbs that have been tested by an independent third party for purity because, unfortunately, many imported Chinese herbs are contaminated. Find out more at www.yinstill.com.

necessary for most women to be restored to full health and build back up her stores of important nutrients such as iron and folate. This advice comes from nutritional research as well as looking at traditional societies. The Mayo Clinic says that families should wait at least 18 months to reduce the risk of complications, such as problems with the placenta, preterm birth, and a low birth-weight baby. There may even be a link between shorter spacing and autism, according to one study that showed that second children were at a greater risk of autism only when the spacing was shorter than three years, and highest when siblings were spaced less than a year. The best spacing in biological terms may be between three and five years. Mayo Clinic research shows that after five years, certain risks such as preterm birth, low birth weight, and preeclampsia go back up. The reason for this isn't known for certain.

Lighting and Fertility

The pineal gland produces the hormone melatonin in response to darkness and uses it to direct all sorts of your body's natural rhythms, including sleep, appetite, and the onset of puberty. The hypothalamus, also located in the brain, regulates the hormonal system and is directly affected by melatonin. Also affected by melatonin are the ovaries and the testes. According to a review of numerous studies published in the journal *Fertility and Sterility*, regular darkness — eight hours every night — is important for both a woman's fertility and for protecting the developing fetus. According to the research, every time you turn on a light — even a very dim light or a screen — it turns down the production of melatonin. Animal studies even suggest a link between behavioural problems in newborns and exposure to excess light in pregnancy, perhaps accounting for ADHD and autism behaviours. Studies also suggest links between disruption of darkness *at night* and obesity, heart disease, diabetes, and even cancer. Blue light — like what comes from screens and obnoxiously bright CFL, LED, and incandescent bulbs — has twice the negative effect on melatonin and the circadian rhythms as other light.

The solution to these effects is simple: don't use your computer close to bedtime, and keep your bedroom nice and dark!

How to Green Your Fertility (for Men and Women)

Here are a series of action steps listed from ♥♥♥ (biggest impact, and possibly more work) to ♥ (quick and easy) to help improve your chances for pregnancy.

1. ♥♥♥ **Assess your overall health.** Remember, fertility is about both partners. What is your daily stress level like? Are you exhausted or depressed? All of these are signs that your body may be under too much strain to

conceive, or, if you do conceive, they may contribute to miscarriage or even developmental disorders in the child. If you are routinely exhausted, fighting depression, struggling with daily tension, having trouble sleeping, or struggling to gain or lose weight, you may be having issues with adrenal fatigue or even hyperthyroidism. The diet suggestions in this book may help, or you may want to seek out the help of a trusted healthcare provider to ensure your thyroid and adrenals are ready for the work of growing and nurturing a baby.

2. ♥♥♥ **Have both partners eat for fertility as you would eat for pregnancy.** First and foremost, go organic. Especially with *all* animal products and oils. (Remember, many toxins — especially those that mess with hormones — concentrate in fats). Know the Dirty Dozen most-contaminated fruits and vegetables and always buy these organic. Learn more in the **Organic-ize Your Diet** section in the Greening Your Pregnancy Diet chapter.

3. ♥♥ **Eat whole foods**, including animal products. The less processed the better. Whole milk is better than skimmed. Broth made from bones is better than bouillon cubes. A bit of wild caught salmon is better than fish sticks. Eat whole grains such as wholegrain sourdough bread. Soak or sprout the grains when possible, such as sprouted quinoa.

4. ♥♥ **Seek out nutrient-dense foods**, like those packed with vitamins A, B, C, D, and E and iodine, zinc, iron, magnesium, folate, essential fatty acids, and antioxidants. These include organic, pastured (or grass-fed for meat) eggs and butter and organ meats, mama-and-baby-safe seafood, beans prepared at home (rather than from a can), and richly coloured (and organic) vegetables such as kale and spinach, cabbages and broccoli, pumpkins, beets, and squash. Sunflowers seeds, flax seeds, raw pumpkin seeds, sesame seeds, almonds, walnuts, olives, garlic, bee pollen, and lentils are all great for fertility. Bone broth from the highest quality animal sources provides gelatin and minerals to the body in preparation for the work of growing a baby. It's easy to make your own: just simmer bones or a carcass for several hours with a bit of apple cider vinegar to help release the nutrients.

5. ♥♥ **Take whole-food-based supplements**, including a very high quality (and mercury-free) version of cod liver or krill oil to help with conception and pregnancy. Read up on all the supplemental advice in the **Greening Your Pregnancy Diet** chapter.

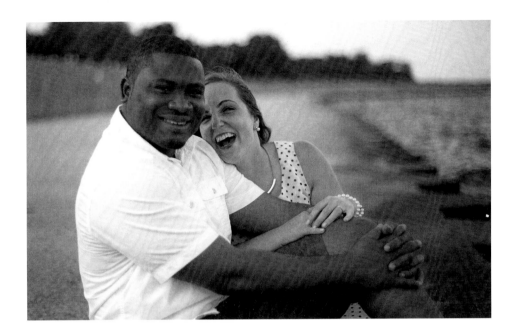

6. ♥♥ **Drink the highest quality water.** Avoid unfiltered tap water and water bottled in plastic. I recommend getting a great water filter that removes chlorine by-products, fluoride, hormones, and pesticides (yes, all of these things can be found in both tap and many bottled waters).

7. ♥♥ **Avoid foods that zap reproductive health:**

- **Refined sugars (especially sugary drinks!) and refined carbohydrates:** The authors of the Harvard Nurse's study, Willett and Chavarro, said that women whose diets had the highest glycemic load — think foods that immediately enter the bloodstream as sugar — were 92 percent more likely to have ovulatory infertility than those whose diets had the lowest glycemic load. This means avoid the sodas, Vitamin Waters, Gatorades, and even pasteurized juices, all of which pack a mean punch to blood sugar levels. As well, avoid the white flour treats. Learn other tips for stabilizing blood sugar in the **Greening Your Pregnancy Diet** chapter.
- **Trans fats:** In a previous study, the same authors found that every 2 percent increase in the consumption of trans fats was associated with a 73 percent increased risk for ovulatory infertility. Trans fats hide in poor quality or partially hydrogenated oils such as Crisco, shortening, and margarine. That means watching out for fried foods (which are almost always fried in partially hydrogenated oils), including fish and chips, French fries, donuts, potato chips, and all those other lovely, greasy favourites.

- **Soy:** As a person who used to eat a lot of soy, I'm sorry to report that soy — especially soy milks and tofu — are full of phytoestrogens that are best avoided by women and men trying to get pregnant and by all children. The phytoestrogens in soy have been shown to negatively affect reproduction and endocrine function and can contribute to thyroid problems (which are linked to infertility and miscarriage). As well, soy can reduce the assimilation of minerals such as calcium, magnesium, copper, and iron and interfere with the body's absorption of vitamins B12 and D and of protein. Men who ate or drank soy were more likely to have lower sperm counts: the equivalent of one cup of soy milk per day was associated with a 50 percent lower sperm count than that of men who didn't eat soy, according to a 2008 study at the Harvard Public School of Health. One study linked a woman's consumption of soy in utero to increased chances of the child developing leukemia, and others with infant boys being born with the male genital disorder hypospadias, although both results may be influenced by the pesticides used in growing soy.
- **Caffeine:** Caffeine was shown to increase the time of conception in otherwise fertile women; women who reported drinking over 300 mg per day of caffeine had a 27 percent lower chance of conceiving for each cycle, according to a study by Hatch and Bracken. As well, a lot of caffeine can disrupt the body's ability to effectively use magnesium, potassium, and calcium, which are particularly important when growing a baby.

8. ♥♥ **Avoid plasticizers** — which are known to mess with hormones — touching or near food. That means to avoid heating or storing foods in plastic storage containers and to be suspicious of the plastic wrap on your cheese and meat (it's full of plasticizers), canned foods, and any foods bought in plastic. Remember that acidic and fatty foods absorb more of the plasticizers than something like pasta.

9. ♥♥ **Care for your microbiome,** so avoid antibiotics unless absolutely necessary, get rid of all those household sources of antibacterial exposure, and eat more fermented foods. I love to make and eat kimchi, sauerkraut, and ginger beer. (See the recipes in the **Green Eating Recipe Handbook** for inspiration.)

10. ♥♥ **Sleep: more and better.** Remember, sleep is one of the only ways to add funds to your adrenal bank account, which helps with all those fertility and growth hormones. To help, especially avoid all screens near bedtime and block out all light — even if you can't sleep — for a full eight hours every night.

11. ♥ Follow all the other amazing advice in this book to help get toxins out of your life.

Conclusion

· ·

Becoming a parent is a time of change, the degree of which is unprecedented in adult lives. The mother's brain — and involved father's — go through more changes than at any other time as adults. The more the brain changes, the easier parenting seems to be. Perhaps this is iconic for all of parenting: the more we are able to give over to the changes involved in parenting, the more our bodies will help. And help is what just about every parent can use. The world is moving faster than ever: new chemicals, new devices, and new worries are emerging faster than we can keep up. Yet our ancient biology is working hard to help us do exactly what we've always done: tune in to our children. In that tuning in, we find hope. Again and again, activists, scientists, and entrepreneurs have described the process of having children as a profound act of hope. Caring for the next generation brings parents, grandparents, and involved citizens together. It is not enough to make decisions that are good enough for today. Holding a new baby in our arms reminds us that we have so much more for which to live.

When I left nonprofit environmental work and started researching, writing, and teaching classes as The Green Mama, I discovered something profound. New parents care. They care about their health, about the environment, and about finding better food and better beauty care products. They care about their homes, their families, and their communities. Now I understand why we care so much. We are preprogrammed to care. Having a baby throws a switch in many of us, and we suddenly feel as if we can no longer put off those changes we know are for the best. We want there to be a better world so that our children don't have to try so hard to become the happy, healthy, and free individuals we know they are destined to be.

As Dr. Bethany Hays, the obstetrician with over 30 years in practice, reminds us, "We don't have babies with our brains." In other words, reading is great (especially if, like me, reading makes you happy), but it's something more primal that births and breastfeeds and guides us into parenting. How can you start to access and foster that part of you?

- **Worry smarter.** As parents we are biologically designed to worry about the obvious dangers: the bear that gets too near our home, the unwashed man on the bus trying to shake hands with our newborn, or the imagined kidnapper lurking around the corner from the playground. Yet in our modern world, these aren't the major threats to our health and happiness. The threats facing us today are very often invisible: they are found in the long list of unpronounceable ingredients in that skin cream, and the dozens of different industrial chemicals added to our foods and smelling up the inside of our homes. As a new parent your brain will help you worry more, so use that worry well. Learn to read labels. Learn to ask better questions of the media, scientists, doctors, and politicians. Is it really proven safe? Who is paying for that study? Why aren't you protecting the health of my children over the economics of a company? How is it possible that this product is so cheap? Is it really as convenient as it is made out to be? Is it really green?

- **Start your new rhythm now.** Kim John Payne, author of *Simplicity Parenting*, reminds parents that we all do better with a gentle rhythm uncluttered by too many activities and strengthened through consistency. In his experience, parents who start before their children are born enjoy the postpartum period more and have an easier adjustment. My first child is what some call "spirited" and others may call "sensitive." I remember reading in Dr. Sears's *The Baby Book* that these children are a blessing that force us to be better parents. It's true. By the time my second came along, I went from a fly-by-the-seat-of-my-pants attitude to an upholder of rhythm. The principles that nurtured my sensitive child and gave me both much-needed time to myself and some predictability include no more than one activity a day (and that might be simply a bath for the first three months), for her to take at least one nap in her bed every day, and a consistent bedtime routine.

- **Let your money be a symbol of your beliefs.** We aren't primarily consumers, we are citizens. Yet most of us spend money, and those dollars tell companies something. If possible, don't tell a company you are willing to buy a product that isn't proven safe, and don't buy from a manufacturer that makes disingenuous claims. Ask yourself, "Will this new thing just be something to trip over in the middle of the night, or will it really help me care for myself and my family better?"

- **Remember, you are what you eat and drink and what you rub on your skin and what you breathe in. And so is your baby.** That principle alone sums up most of this book. When overwhelmed or confused by choices, this will help set you straight. If I am still confused, I usually think about my great-grandmother and what she would do.

- **Birth matters.** Not many people are likely to get exactly the birth they imagine. Yet research into what physiological birth looks like will help you imagine it more clearly and help you get a healthier birth with fewer interventions. Birth is both an ending and a beginning; everybody is happier when that transition is without trauma.

- **The postpartum period deserves pre-planning.** The more support and the less activity you have planned for the postpartum period, the better. Gather supplies beforehand and prepare to be pampered. Remember, no matter how much you love and want that baby, almost every mother will also struggle a bit during this time. The hormones and brain are going through tremendous transformation. You barely get any sleep. Everything is new, and it all seems to matter so, so much. It helps just to know that feeling all of this simply makes you human. It also helps if you take your cod liver oil and prenatal vitamins, and eat really nutritious food. Anytime you can sleep, sleep. Anything you can do lying down, do lying down. Anything that can be done sitting, sit. This is a time for recovery, not for getting back into those pre-pregnancy jeans. If you are so exhausted or depressed that you can't do *anything* or if you have violent thoughts toward your child or yourself, these are signs that you would benefit from help from a medical professional with experience in postpartum depression. Postpartum depression is extremely common, so please don't add shame to your list of burdens, and get the help you need.

- **Do less and do what you love.** There are so many worthwhile causes in which to get involved. There are so many activities for pregnant women, and even more for new parents and when your children get older. What to do? It might benefit you to know that there isn't research to suggest that those really early lessons and classes benefit children in the ways that really matter: they aren't smarter, happier, or even better socialized in the long run because they took baby ballet or infant music. Instead, do fewer things and prioritize your happiness and things you can do together. The research suggests that less frazzled mothers are happier mothers and happier mothers have happier children. I loved being with other new mamas who shared common interests after having my first baby. I loved leading Green Mama Cafes with new moms to discuss greening parenthood. I loved going door-to-door before an election with my baby strapped to my chest. But I didn't love those bitchy and fear-inducing new-mom chat groups online and I didn't love dragging my newborn to her older sister's two-hour, three-days-a-week preschool. In hindsight I wish I would have skipped the latter stuff.

- **Learn techniques to de-stress.** Stress isn't just something in your mind, and it isn't just something you are (or aren't) doing. Stress is strain, and it comes from the toxins in our environment, poor food, traffic, pollution, technology, and the stories that we tell ourselves. Our bodies will work better to digest that food, manage those toxins, and recover from the jerk cutting you off on the way to work if you have a way to relax. Try meditation, yoga, walking in nature, reading, doing jigsaw puzzles, colouring, painting, or taking warm (but not too hot when you're pregnant) baths. All of these have proven de-stressing benefits! Don't stop after you have the baby. Having a baby is stress-producing in the best of situations: hormones are fluctuating, the brain is changing rapidly, and you have to learn everything there is to know about a new being (or two). Give yourself a break! Literally, give yourself a brea*k every day.* Your baby won't "break" if you leave her to sleep — or even cry — while you take a mental health minute (or fifteen). My sanity-saving activity when I was home with a newborn was scalding hot baths with Epsom salts: *Ahhhhh!*

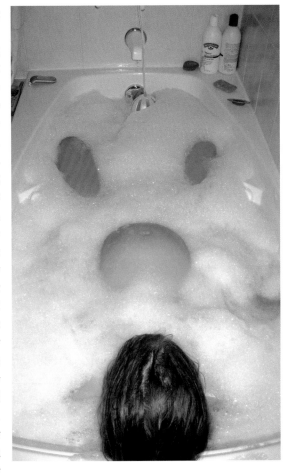

- **Create community locally.** Start a playgroup or host a play date. Share green tips, babysitting duties, and meals. It will be easier to stay on your path if you don't feel alone. And there are neurological benefits from being in community with other like-minded people.

- **Be proactive.** Take that minute to write or make a phone call to your political representative or a company about a product. Politicians act on what they hear their constituents demanding (and sometimes the other "side" is quite loud); companies can change dramatically if they know it matters to their customers. Even if the change you want doesn't happen right away, just doing it makes it easier for you to do it the next time and sets an example for your child. Perhaps your playgroup will be just as interested as you in what you're learning. Did you know in Canada you can send a postcard or letter with your concerns or kudos to the governor general, any member of the Senate and House of Commons, or the prime minister for free (no postage required)?

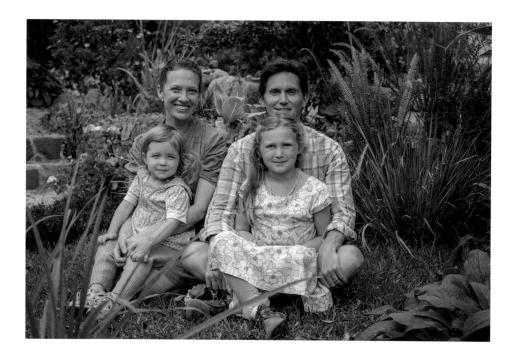

- **Laugh and play more.** Laughing is really good medicine for pregnant women, postpartum women, and children. What is your form of play? Online anything doesn't count because the research suggests that it can rewire your brain, and not in a good way. Learn how to play for real, and teach your child that life is also fun.

Acknowledgements

· ·

Am I the only person in the world that reads acknowledgements (I mean the ones you know you aren't likely to be in)? Just in case I'm not, I'll keep it short. Just like a person is multi-faceted, so is any book. I am grateful to all the people and talents that helped make this book happen. In my children's school we say education is the work of the head, hands, and heart. This book, which I hope will educate and inspire you, represents a great deal of generosity from others that shared in all three areas.

Thank you to the Head. By that I mean all of those scientists, researchers, entrepreneurs, and health experts who toil to give us a greater understanding of ourselves and our world. It is humbling, awesome, and inspiring work. Some of the heady-folks that gave graciously to the creation of this book include Dr. Bruce Lanphear, Dr. Bethany Hays, Margaret Floyd Barry, Kate Koyote, Dr. Spence Pentland, Dr. Katie Dahlgren, Paul Hawken, Kim John Payne, Jennifer Block, Susun Weed, Geraldine Matus, Maggie MacDonald, Rick Smith, Ralph Danyluk, Heather Gibson, Sonya McLeod, Jem Terra, Jingo Lewis, Summer Knight, Insiya Rasiwala-Finn, and Cassie Rodgers. I am also thankful to all the many green mamas and The Green Mama helpers who have given some of their life energy to bringing their own experiences, inspiration, and research to the world.

Thank you to the Hands. Writing is a craft and it takes practice and guidance. For this, I am most thankful to my readers, editors, agents, and publishers. This includes the magical and mighty Cary Saxifrage, the indomitable Chris Cassucio as well as Hilary McMahon and the entire gang at Westwood Creative Artists, and my lovely team at Dundurn publishing, including the amazing editorial team that helped with my book — Allison Hirst, Kathryn Lane, and the "Jennys" — and the many other talented folks that helped with all those behind-the-scenes details from art and layout to marketing and distribution, in particular Margaret Bryant and Jaclyn Hodsdon.

The hands also hold cameras. The photography time and talent that goes into the creation of the Green Mama books is a tremendous work of creativity, love, and generosity. Thank you for this Vanessa Zises Filley, Roxanne Engstrom, and Cassie Rodgers.

Thank you as well to *EcoParent Magazine* for permission to reprint an earlier version of the Green Baby Shower Handbook that I had previously published in their wonderful magazine; to Susan Weed for allowing me to reprint her incredible recipes; and to Bruce Lanphear and Little Things Matter Productions for the use of their graph on page 81.

Thank you to the Heart. The more I learn about life, health, and the art of parenting, the more grateful I am to my family of origin and my family of creation. I am so grateful to my ancestors for all they did to make my life possible, especially my grandmothers Rose Gillespie and Ethel Mae Hansen. My grandma Ethel Mae died during the writing of this second book, but her wisdom continues to influence how I look at the act of parenting and the art of home-making. Thank you to my mom, Karen, for that loving womb and for generally being such an inspiration of how to gently question the status quo. Thank you to my dad, Mike, for all that healthy sperm and for gifting me with your whole-hearted smile. A special thanks to my siblings — and my in-laws, in-loves, steps, and D.G.s — for teaching me that love is not born of genetics. A special thanks to my sister Tosha, who kindly got pregnant and had a baby while I was writing this book so that I could be reminded of all the details involved in the hard work of growing life.

I thank my lucky stars everyday that I somehow managed to marry and stay married to the world's most awesome man. I love you Sadhu and I thank you for helping give me the world's two most interesting and loveable children. Thank you Zella Rose and Maela for choosing me. I love being your mama with my whole self: head, hands, and heart.

Green Mama-to-Beware

· ·

The ABCs: Avoid These "Bad" Chemicals When You're Pregnant
Here's what you need to know about the most common toxins that we know are best to avoid as much as possible in pregnancy.

Heavy Metals

Of the heavy metals, arsenic, lead, and mercury are three of the most prevalent and are highly toxic, persist in the environment for many years, and can bio-accumulate (be stored) in our bodies. There are no safe levels. The research suggests that most, perhaps all, heavy metals pass through the placental barrier and can be detrimental to the growing fetus, permanently damaging organs and brain development. Studies have found mercury at double the concentrations in the baby's cord blood compared to the mother. Arsenic has been found at about 80 percent concentrations in the baby's cord blood. The other heavy metals — lead, cobalt, and selenium — seem to be somewhat more filtered by the placenta.

Arsenic can be naturally forming, but the one to watch out for is the inorganic version, which enters the environment from treated lumber, coal-fired power plants, and arsenical pesticide runoff. The latter has contributed to groundwater contamination and is the suspected source of the high levels of arsenic found in rice. Rice is now considered the highest food source of arsenic exposure for most people, especially babies who, relative to body weight, consume three times more rice than adults, primarily in the form of infant rice cereal. Arsenic is known to cause cancer (in other words, it's carcinogenic), and recent testing by the FDA shows that pregnant mothers who eat more rice may have children with decreased learning performances.

Lead exposure has been linked with hyperactivity, lower IQs, and neurocognitive disorders such as ADHD; can damage kidneys, blood, muscles, and bones; and is likely carcinogenic. While lead is still found in 100 percent of babies born today, our exposure has decreased thanks to environmental regulations on coal burning, emissions, and the use of lead in consumer products such as paint and gasoline.

Mercury is a particular risk to babies-to-be and children. As with many heavy metals, small amounts of mercury occur naturally in the environment, but there is no known safe level or any use for it in our bodies. Instead, it poses a risk to a child's developing brain, neurological system, and organs, and any amount can cause permanent damage. The good news is that by far the greatest human exposures to mercury come from man-made activities, such as coal-burning power plants, the healthcare sector, mining, and charcoal production. Because these sources are man-made, they can be regulated and improved. The greatest source of mercury exposure for most children is from fish, but they can also be exposed to significant sources from rice and medical products, such as amalgam fillings. These exposures are likely to be to methyl mercury, the most studied, and thus considered the most toxic form of mercury. Children can also be exposed to the less studied ethyl mercury from multi-dose vaccines. In Canada that might include the multi-dose flu vaccine, the tetanus toxoid vaccine, and the hepatitis B vaccine.

Persistent Organic Pollutants (POPs)

POPs are toxic chemicals that travel on wind and water and accumulate in the bodies of animals. They have found their way into the haze surrounding the Arctic and the polar bears, as well as into your unborn child, and they will likely find their way into your future grandchildren because they are readily passed across the placenta and stick around for a long time. POPs travel easily and far and don't pay attention to international borders. Indeed, many accumulate in remote, seemingly pristine places like the polar regions and the Arctic, where they get stuck because of the wind patterns and the cold. Small amounts can cause big problems, including brain changes that can manifest in learning disabilities, ADHD, autism, thyroid problems, hormonal disruption, and cancer. Canada and more than 90 other countries regulate the 12 most dangerous POPs — including furans and dioxins — as part of the 2014 Stockholm Convention. The good news is that the POPs targeted under the original 1972 agreement, including DDT and PCBs, have been substantially reduced in the environment and in humans (although many of them, such as PCBs, are still found in nearly 100 percent of newborns). Unfortunately, there are still only 12 POPs targeted under the 2014 agreement, and many additional POPs are out there and new ones are being created.

Dioxin and certain pesticides are POPs, those nonstick substances on your frying pan are POPs, and so are those chemical flame retardants in your child's foam mattress.

Chemical flame retardants to watch out for include brominated flame retardants (PBDEs) and the phosphate esters (Tris), including TDCP and TCEP phosphate. All three have been linked to serious health problems, including neurological disorders, hormonal disruption, organ damage, thyroid disorders, and fertility problems, and may be linked to cancer. Young children are still one of the groups most highly exposed to Tris flame retardants, although it was banned in 1977 from children's sleepwear when it was discovered to mutate children's DNA. PBDE levels are 75 times higher in American women than their European counterparts, likely because of a California law requiring flame retardancy for items sold in that state. Both the United States and Health Canada have asked manufacturers to phase out certain PBDE compounds, but PBDE — as well as Tris — are still on the market and common in children's products. As well, many of the new chemical flame retardants on the market to replace them are thought to be just as bad, but are less tested.

Perfluorinated compounds (PFCs) are used to make things stain-, oil-, or water-resistant. They are used in stain guards to magically keep red wine from staining your white couch, make cookware nonstick, and make clothing waterproof. PFCs are also used in grease-resistant food packaging such as hamburger wrappers, chip bags, and microwave popcorn packages. They can even coat your dental floss. Two of the most infamous are PFOA and PFOS. Both have been found in nearly every human studied, and levels in children are often higher than in adults. PFCs have been linked to cancer and birth defects. Because of the known health concerns associated with PFOA and PFOS, they are mostly being phased out in the United States and Canada, but it's best to beware of the alternatives for now as well.

Dioxin is formed as an unintended by-product of many industrial processes involving chlorine, including the manufacturing of pesticides, the production and incineration of PVC plastics, and paper bleaching. Polychlorinated biphenyls (PCBs) are dioxin-like compounds that, unlike most dioxins, are intentionally produced for use in electrical insulators, fire-fighting compounds, paint, lubricants, and transformer fluid. Dioxin and its relatives are often referred to as super-toxins, and the IARC considers the most potent dioxins to be Group 1 carcinogens. They are linked to birth defects, infertility, reduced sperm counts, endometriosis, diabetes, learning disabilities, immune system suppression, lung problems, skin disorders, and numerous cancers. Traces of dioxins can be found in air, water, and soil, and —

from there — they work their way up the food chain and into the fat of fish, animals, and humans. Diet, particularly meat and dairy, is considered our primary source of exposure.

Pesticides make up the majority of the POPS restricted under the Stockholm Convention. Nevertheless, pesticides such as DDT continue to be freely used in much of the developing world despite the known disastrous effects on human health and their ability to travel freely across the globe. Many newer pesticides are less persistent, but just as pervasive. For example, glyphosate is found in Round-Up, the world's most commonly used agricultural pesticide and the second most-applied residential pesticide in the United States. Glyphosate is linked to miscarriage, reproductive damage, and ADHD, and animal studies show that it has the ability to alter genes.

Volatile Organic Compounds (VOCs)

VOCs include a wide range of carbon-based chemicals that easily vaporize (off-gas) from numerous household and workplace sources. VOCs can cause immediate health issues, such as headaches, and numerous VOCs are linked to neurological and organ damage, chemical sensitivities, and cancer. Pregnant women are especially vulnerable, as studies have suggested that increased exposure is directly linked to lower neurological function in their offspring. VOC exposures are also linked to miscarriage and congenital malformations. VOCs react quickly, and concentrations will usually decrease over time. Examples of VOCs include formaldehyde, phthalates, gasoline, benzene, and solvents including toluene, xylene, styrene, and perchloroethylene (PERC), used in dry cleaning. Many VOCs, such as those found in cosmetic products, furniture, paints, and cleaning items, have an odour, and the "sniff test" can alert you to their presence. Women can be exposed to VOCs at work — in dry cleaners, photography studios, and nail or hair salons — and at home — from pressed-wood furniture, paints, air fresheners, copiers or printers, cigarette smoke, and other petroleum-based products.

Formaldehyde is a smelly, colourless, flammable VOC classified as a Group 1 carcinogen by the IARC. It is known to cause cancer in humans and animals. It can irritate the eyes, nose, and throat and trigger asthma. Formaldehyde can be found in furniture and toys and anything else made of pressed wood or particle board. It can also be found in some glues, such as those used in hanging wallpaper or laying carpet, and it is a by-product released from as much as one-third of all cosmetics, such as shampoos — even those marketed to children. Emissions from furniture generally decrease over time (in other words, are off-gassed), but it can take as much as seven years just to reach minimal levels. Unfortunately, the let-it-get-old method of harm reduction doesn't apply to everything that may contain formaldehyde. Old shampoo isn't any safer than the new stuff.

Phthalates are VOCs and plasticizers found primarily in cosmetics and plastics. They are considered likely hormone mimickers and have been linked to preterm birth, infertility, and cancer. A CDC study found 75 percent of participants had detectible levels of phthalates in their bodies. The six phthalates considered most hazardous have been banned in the EU since 1999. The United States and Canada have also banned *some* phthalates in *some* children's products and toys, but not in personal care products.

Benzene, toluene, ethylbenzene, and xylene can be found individually or together, referred to as BTEX, and can contaminate air, soil, and water. They range from known (benzene) to suspected human carcinogens. They can pass through breast milk and through the placenta. Some have been found to accumulate in a woman's breast tissue. They are routinely found in petroleum by-products, and all or some can be found in solvents, paints, nail polish, hair dyes, some cleaning products, and cosmetics.

Toxic Plastics

Plastics are everywhere. They can do amazing things, but unfortunately many, if not most, of them come with some big health costs, including exposing us to chemicals that mimic estrogen. Some of the worst offenders include the following:

PVC, or vinyl, contains lead and phthalates, and releases dioxin. It is linked to neurotoxic effects and endocrine problems. It is found in soft, pliable plastic products like crib mattress covers and shower curtains and in vinyl blinds and siding.

Bisphenol-containing compounds including BPA and BPS and 38 other known or suspected endocrine disruptors contain bisphenol. BPA may cause problems of brain and hormone development, decreased sperm counts, erectile dysfunction, heart disease, diabetes, liver abnormalities, and breast cancer. BPS can disrupt a cell's normal functioning and may lead to diabetes and obesity, asthma, birth defects, and cancer. Bisphenol-containing compounds, including BPA itself, can be found in hard plastic items, such as your water bottles and baby bottles, and in the lining of canned goods, including baby formula, even in ones labelled BPA-free.

Melamine is a chemical by-product of industrial processes and is added to some plastics (and some foods, such as in the baby formula scandal). It is linked to kidney failure. Melamine products may also release the toxin formaldehyde. It is found in many children's plates and cups that are sold as "BPA-free" or "shatterproof" and it looks like hard plastic.

Polystyrene, or **Styrofoam**, contains the toxic substances styrene and benzene, suspected carcinogens and neurotoxins that are hazardous to humans. Hot foods and liquids, alcohol, oils, acidic foods, and red wine can cause Styrofoam to release toxins into the food or drink.

Twenty Concerning Cosmetic Ingredients

1. **Aluminum** is a known neurotoxin that serves no purpose in any amount in the body and is hiding out in your antiperspirant as well as some toothpaste.
2. **BHA** and **BHT** have been linked to aquatic toxicity and liver, kidney, and thyroid problems, and may promote tumour growth and mimic estrogen. They can be found as preservatives in cosmetics. Look for *butylated hydroxyanisole* or *butylated hydroxytoluene*.
3. **Boric acid** can interfere with hormones and cause lower sperm counts and male infertility. They can be found in diaper creams. Look as well for *sodium borate* or *hydrogen borate*.
4. **Coal tar dyes** can cause cancer in humans. Look for p-phenylenediamine, paraphenylenediamine, or 1,4-benzenediamine, and colours listed as *"CI"* followed by a five-digit number. For U.S. products, look for *FD&C* followed by a colour name.
5. **DEET** is a suspected neurotoxin used primarily to kill mosquitoes. Its overuse — even topically — has resulted in death. Look for *N,N-Diethyl-meta-toluamide*.
6. **Dioxane**-containing ingredients can be contaminated with 1,4-dioxane, linked to cancer. Look on the label for words ending in *-eth*, *SLS*, *sodium lauryl sulfate*, or *PEG*.
7. **Dioxins** are considered a super (and we don't mean in a good way) toxin. They find their way into bleached tampons (which are all tampons that aren't organic and unbleached) and into bleached diapers.
8. **Ethanolamines** are suspected carcinogens, can damage organs, and cause allergies. They can react with other chemicals in cosmetics to form carcinogenic nitrosamines, which are regulated under the Hotlist, but not when they occur unintentionally. They are found in makeup, perfumes, sunscreens, hair care, lotions, and soaps. Look for *MEA*, *DEA*, *TEA*, and numerous variations such as *cocamide DEA*, *Triethanolamine*, *diethanolamine*, and *TEA-lauryl sulfate*.

9. **Formaldehyde** is a known human carcinogen. It can be found in eyelash glue and in hair smoothing and straightening applications (beware the Brazilian Blowout, for instance). Formaldehyde can also be released from preservatives such as *bronopol, bronidox, 5-bromo-5-nitro-1,3-dioxane, Diazolidinyl Urea, DMDM hydantoin, Hydroxymethylglycinate, Imidazolidinyl urea, Quaternium-15,* and *Tris (hydroxymethyl) nitromethane.*

10. **Fragrance, perfume**, or **parfum** can include a mixture of dozens or hundreds of ingredients, even in cosmetics labelled *unscented.* Fragrances can trigger or even cause allergies and asthma, and some are known or suspected carcinogens or neurotoxins or are harmful to wildlife.

11. **Heavy metals,** including lead, arsenic, mercury, aluminum, zinc, chromium, and iron, are found in a variety of cosmetics, including lipstick, mascara, whitening toothpaste, eyeliner, nail colour, foundations, eye shadows, blush, concealers, and antiperspirants. Heavy metals have been linked to reproductive, immune, and nervous system toxicity, as well as brain damage. Heavy metals can pass into a fetus. Unfortunately, heavy metals often don't appear on a label at all, but can show up as *calmel, lead acetate, mercurio, mercuric, mercurochrome,* and *thimerosal.*

12. **Iodopropynyl butylcarbamate** is a preservative suspected to cause human reproductive and developmental issues, possible infertility, problems in pregnancy, and birth defects. It can be found in many kinds of cosmetics, including cream, lotion, concealer, eyeshadow, mascara, shampoo, and more. Look out for *IBP, IPBC, butyl-3-iodo-2 propynylcarbamate, carbamic acid, Glycacil,* and *IODOCARB.*

13. **Oxybenzone** and other chemical sunscreens can mimic hormones and cause allergies. They are used in sunscreens and some UV-protecting moisturizers. Look out for words that include *benzone* and *octinoxate.* Opt for non-nanoparticle mineral sunscreens instead.

14. **Parabens** are chemical preservatives used in cosmetics that may be linked to cancer, developmental disorders, and hormonal issues. Look out for words with *paraben* or *p-hydroxybenzoic acid esters.*

15. **Petroleum distillates** or petroleum-containing compounds can be contaminated with polycrylic aromatic hydrocarbons or other impurities from the oil-refining process that may cause cancer. Look out for *petrolatum, mineral oil,* and *petroleum jelly.*

16. **Phenoxyethanol** is another chemical preservative linked to reproductive issues and nervous system and brain damage. Also look for the name *ethylene glycol mophenyl ether.*

17. **Phthalates** can be used in cosmetics as plasticizers, fixatives, or solvents and are suspected endocrine disruptors and reproductive toxicants. Look for ingredients that end in *phthalate, DBP, DMP, DEP,* or *fragrance.*

18. **Siloxanes** are suspected endocrine disruptors and reproductive toxicants and are harmful to fish and other wildlife. They are used in cosmetics such as moisturizers, facial treatments, and some deodorants. Look for *-siloxane* or *-methicone* in the ingredient list.

19. **Toluene** and **benzene** are toxins linked to cancer and neurological issues. They can end up in such things as dyes, glues, paints, and paint thinners and such cosmetics as hair dye, coloured cosmetics, and fingernail polish and remover. Look for *benzene, methylbenzene, phenylmethane,* or *toluol.*

20. **Triclosan** is a pesticide linked to endocrine disruption and antibiotic resistance. It can be found in toothpaste, antiperspirants, and the majority of hand soaps. Look for anything labelled *antibacterial* or the ingredient *Microban.*

Further Reading

● ●

The Baby Book by William and Martha Sears

Being Fertile by Dr. Spence Pentland

Birthing from Within: An Extra-Ordinary Guide to Childbirth Preparation by
    Pam England

Blessed Unrest and other books by Paul Hawken

Cure Your Child with Food by Kelly Dorfman

Eat Naked book and cookbook by Margaret Floyd Barry

Ecoholic series of books by Adria Vasil

Green Mama: Giving Your Child a Healthy Start and a Greener Future by
    Manda Aufochs Gillespie

Having Faith and *Raising Elijah* by Sandra Steingraber

Healthy Sleep Habits, Happy Child by Marc Weissbluth

Homeopathic Medicine at Home by Maesimun Panos and Jane Heimlich

Husband-Coached Childbirth: The Bradley Method of Natural Childbirth by
    Robert Bradley and Ashley Montagu

Ina May's Guide series by Ina May Gaskin

A Natural Guide to Pregnancy and Postpartum Health by Dean Raffelock,
    Robert Rountree, and Virginia Hopkins

Nourishing Traditions series by Sally Fallon Morell

The Pregnancy Journal by A. Christine Harris

Pushed: The Painful Truth About Childbirth and Modern Maternity Care and
    Below the Belt by Jennifer Block

Real Food series by Nina Planck (includes how to eat during pregnancy and
    while breastfeeding)

Rebuild from Depression: A Nutrient Guide by Amanda Rose

Resource for Informed Breastmilk Sharing by Maria Armstrong and Shell Walker

Simplicity Parenting by Kim John Payne

Slow Death by Rubber Duck and *ToxIn, ToxOut* by Rick Smith and Bruce Lourie
Taking Charge of Your Fertility by Toni Weschler
The Thinking Woman's Guide to a Better Birth by Henci Goer
Wise Woman Herbal for the Childbearing Year and other books by Susun Weed
The Womanly Art of Breastfeeding by La Leche League International
Vaccinations: A Thoughtful Parent's Guide and other books by Aviva Jill Romm

Online resources

www.aborm.org
www.adriavasil.com
www.anandawithin.com
www.babylist.com
www.bestforbabes.org
www.bfmed.org
www.breastfeedingcanada.ca
www.breastfeedinginc.ca
www.buildinggreen.com
www.cagbc.org
www.canadianbreastfeedingfoundation.org
www.cornucopia.org
www.davidsuzuki.org
www.eatnakednow.com
www.eatsonfeets.org
www.ecoparent.ca
www.ehatlas.ca
environmentaldefence.ca
www.evergreen.ca
www.ewg.org
www.functionalmedicine.org
www.thegreenmama.com
hbelc.org
www.healthychild.org
www.healthyenvironmentforkids.ca
www.thehealthyhomeeconomist.com
www.holistichealingarts.org
www.hm4hb.net
inbedorganics.com

www.ican-online.org
www.infactcanada.ca
www.infantrisk.com
www.jenniferblock.com
www.justisse.ca
www.kellymom.com
www.klinghardtacademy.com
www.theleakyboob.com
lifewithoutplastic.com
www.littlemountainhomeopathy.com
www.lllc.ca
www.lllusa.org
www.matraea.com
www.mothering.com
www.motherisk.com
www.myhealthempowered.com
neitra.ca
www.neufeldinstitute.org
www.organicconsumers.org
www.paulhawken.com
www.rainestudy.org.au
sokindregistry.org
www.susunweed.com
toxnet.nlm.nih.gov
well.ca
www.westonaprice.org
www.whatsonmyfood.org
www.yinstill.com
www.yogue.ca

Sources

• •

Chapter 1: Greening the Womb

Belluck, Pam. "In Study, Fatherhood Leads to Drop in Testosterone." *New York Times*, September 12, 2011.

Borreli, Lizette. "The Science Behind 'Pregnancy Brain': Why Pregnant Women Experience Grey Matter Loss, Neurological Changes." *Medical Daily*, December 19, 2016. www.medicaldaily.com/science-behind-pregnancy-brain-why-pregnant-women-experience-grey-matter-loss-406765.

Curley, J.P., R. Mashoodh, and F.A. Champagne. "Epigenetics and the Origins of Paternal Effects." *Hormones and Behaviours* 59, no. 3 (2011): 306–14. doi:10.1016/j.yhbeh.2010.06.018.

Environmental Health Atlas. www.ehatlas.ca.

Gettler, Lee, Thomas McDade, Alan Feranil, et al. "Longitudinal Evidence that Fatherhood Decreases Testosterone in Human Males." *Proceedings of the National Academy of Sciences* 108, no. 39 (2011): 16194–99. doi:10.1073/pnas.1105403108.

Kim, Pilyoung, James F. Leckman, Linda C. Mayes, et al. "The Plasticity of Human Maternal Brain: Longitudinal Changes in Brain Anatomy During the Early Postpartum Period." *Behavioural Neuroscience* 124, no. 5 (2010): 695–700. doi:10.1037/a0020884.

Lafrance, Adrienne. "What Happens to a Woman's Brain When She Becomes a Mother." *Atlantic*, January 8, 2015.

Mossop, Brian. "The Science of Fatherhood." *Scientific American Mind*, July 2011.

Mueller, N.T., et al. "The Infant Microbiome Development: Mom Matters." *Trends in Molecular Medicine* 21, no. 2 (2015): 109–17. doi:10.1016/j.molmed.2014.12.002.

National Institutes of Health. "NIH Human Microbiome Project Defines Normal Bacterial Makeup of the Body." *NIH*, June 13, 2012. www.nih. gov/news/health/jun2012/nhgri-13.htm. Accessed February 23, 2014.

President's Cancer Panel. "Reducing Environmental Cancer Risk: What We Can Do Now." *2008–2009 Annual Report*. 2010.

Public Health Agency of Canada. "Thimerosol-Updated Statement." Canada Communicable Disease Report, National Advisory Committee on Immunization. Volume 33, July 2007. www.phac-aspc.gc.ca.

Schapiro, Mark. "Toxic Inaction: Why Poisonous, Unregulated Chemicals End Up in Our Blood." *Harper's Magazine*, October 2007.

Skakkebaek, N.E., E. Rajpert-De Meyts, and K.M. Main. "Testicular Dysgenesis Syndrome: An Increasingly Common Developmental Disorder with Environmental Aspects: Opinion" *Human Reproduction* 16, no. 5 (2001): 972–78. doi:10.1093/humrep/16.5.972.

Chapter 2: Greening Your Pregnancy Diet and The Green Eating Recipe Handbook

Aasheim, Erlend T., et al. "Vitamin Status in Morbidly Obese Patients: A Cross-Sectional Study," *American Journal of Clinical Nutrition* 87, no. 2 (2008): 362–69.

Adams, K.M., M. Kohlmeier, and S.H. Zeisel. "Nutrition Education in U.S. Medical Schools: Latest Update of a National Survey." *Academic Medicine: Journal of the Association of American Medical Colleges* 85, no. 9 (2010): 1537–42. doi:10.1097/ACM.0b013e3181eab71b.

Aris, Aziz, and Samuel Leblanc. "Maternal and Fetal Exposure to Pesticides Associated to Genetically Modified Foods in Eastern Townships of Quebec, Canada." *Reproductive Toxicology* 31, no. 4 (2011): 528–33.

Axon, A., et al. "Tartrazine and Sunset Yellow are Xenoestrogens in a New Screening Assay to Identify Modulators of Human Oestrogen Receptor Transcriptional Activity." *Toxicology* 298, no. 1–3 (2012): 40–51. doi:10.1016/j.tox.2012.04.014.

Barker, D.J.P. "The Origins of the Developmental Origins Theory." *Journal of Internal Medicine* 261 (2007): 412–17. doi:10.1111/j.1365-2796.2007.01809.x.

Bateman B., J.O. Warner, E. Hutchinson, et al. "The Effects of a Double Blind, Placebo Controlled, Artificial Food Colourings and Benzoate Preservative Challenge on Hyperactivity in a General Population Sample of Preschool Children." *Archives of Disease in Childhood* 89 (2004): 506–11.

Belpoggi, F., et al. "Results of Long-Term Carcinogenicity Bioassay on Sprague-Dawley Rats Exposed to Aspartame Administered in Feed." *Annals of the New York Academy of Sciences* 1076 (2006): 559–77.

Benbrook, Charles M., et al. "New Evidence Confirms the Nutritional Superiority of Plant-Based Organic Foods." *Organic Center*, March 2008.

Berg, J.M., J.L. Tymoczko, and L. Stryer. *Biochemistry*, 5th edition. New York: W H Freeman, 2002. Section 8.6, "Vitamins Are Often Precursors to Coenzymes." www.ncbi.nlm.nih.gov/books/NBK22549.

Blot, W.J., B.E. Henderson, and J.D. Boice Jr. "Childhood Cancer in Relation to Cured Meat Intake: Review of the Epidemiological Evidence." *Nutrition and Cancer* 34, no. 1 (1999): 111–18.

Botta, Amy, and Sanjoy Ghosh. "Exploring the Impact of n-6 PUFA-rich Oilseed Production on Commercial Butter Compositions Worldwide." *Journal of Agricultural and Food Chemistry* (2016). doi:10.1021/acs.jafc.6b03353.

Bunin, G.R., et al. "Maternal Diet and Risk of Astrocytic Glioma in Children: A Report from the Childrens Cancer Group (United States and Canada)." *Cancer Causes Control* 5, no. 2 (1994): 177–87.

Canadian Biotechnology Action Network. "Report 1: Where in the World Are GM Crops and Foods?" March 19, 2015.

Catalano, P.M. et al. "Fetuses of Obese Mothers Develop Insulin Resistance in Utero." *Diabetes Care* 32, no. 6 (2009): 1076–80.

"Chicken and Egg Page." *Mother Earth News.* www.motherearthnews.com/homesteading-and-livestock/eggs-zl0z0703zswa.

Coletta, J.M., S.J. Bell, and A.S. Roman. "Omega-3 Fatty Acids and Pregnancy." *Reviews in Obstetrics and Gynecology* 3, no. 4 (2010): 163–71.

Coyle, J.T. "Glutamate Receptors and Age-Related Neurodegenerative Disorders." *Biological Psychiatry* 27, no. 91A (1990).

Craig-Schmidt, M.C. "Isomeric Fatty Acids: Evaluating Status and Implications for Maternal and Child Health." *Lipids* 36, no. 9 (2001): 997–1006.

Dhaka, V., et al. "Trans Fats: Sources, Health Risks and Alternative Approach — A Review." *Journal of Food Science and Technology* 48, no. 5 (2011): 534–41. doi:10.1007/s13197-010-0225-8.

Dietrich, M., et al. "A Review: Dietary and Endogenously Formed N-Nitroso Compounds and Risk of Childhood Brain Tumors." *Cancer Causes and Control* 16, no. 6 (2005): 619–35.

Domar, Alice D., and Sheila Curry Oakes. *Finding Calm for the Expectant Mom: Tools for Reducing Stress, Anxiety, and Mood Swings During Your Pregnancy.* New York: Penguin Random House, 2016.

Dunsworth, Holly M., et al. "Metabolic Hypothesis for Human Altriciality."

Proceedings of the National Academy of Sciences 109, no. 38 (2012): 15212–216. doi:10.1073/pnas.1205282109.

Fallon, Sally, and Mary G. Enig. *Nourishing Traditions: The Cookbook That Challenges Politically Correct Nutrition and the Diet Dictocrats.* Washington, DC: New Trends, 2001.

Forman Cody, Lisa. "Eating for Two: Shaping Mothers' Figures and Babies' Futures in Modern American Culture." *Gender, Health, and Popular Culture: Historical Perspectives.* Ed. Cheryl Kranick Warsh. Waterloo, ON: Wilfrid Laurier University Press, 2011.

González, Piñero, et al. "Organochlorine Pesticide Residues in Four Types of Vegetable Oils." *Archivos Latinoamericanos de Nutrición* 57, no. 4 (2007): 397–401.

Gunier, Robert B., et al. "Prenatal Residential Proximity to Agricultural Pesticide Use and IQ in 7-Year-Old Children." *Environmental Health Perspectives* (2016). doi:10.1289/EHP504.

Gunnars, Kris, "How to Optimize Your Omega-6 to Omega-3 Ratio." *Authority Nutrition.* https://authoritynutrition.com/optimize-omega-6-omega-3-ratio. Accessed December 28, 2016.

Hites, Ronald A., et al. "Global Assessment of Organic Contaminants in Farmed Salmon." *Science* 303, no. 5655 (2004): 226–29.

Holford, Patrick. *Optimum Nutrition for the Mind.* London: Hachette Digital, 2007.

Hollis, B.W., et al. "Vitamin D Supplementation During Pregnancy: Double-Blind, Randomized Clinical Trial of Safety and Effectiveness." *Journal of Bone and Mineral Research* 26, no. 10 (2011): 2341–57. doi:10.1002/jbmr.463.

"How We Got Here: The Barker Hypothesis and the Developmental Origins of Health and Disease." *Better the Future.* http://betterthefuture.org/how-we-got-here-the-barker-hypothesis-and-the-developmental-origins-of-health-and-disease.

Kidd, Paris. "An Approach to the Nutritional Management of Autism." *Alternative Therapies* 9, no. 5 (2003).

Koletzko, B. "Supply, Metabolism and Biological Effects of Trans-isomeric Fatty Acids in Infants." [Article in German] *Nahrung* 35, no. 3 (1991): 229–83.

Larson, S.C., and A. Wolk. "Red and Processed Meat Consumption and Risk of Pancreatic Cancer: Meta-Analysis of Prospective Studies." *British Journal of Cancer* 104 (2012): 1196–201. doi:10.1038/ bjc.2011.58.

Lorden, J.F., and A. Claudle. "Behavioral and Endocrinological Effects of Single Injections of Monosodium Glutamate in the Mouse." *Neuro-behavioral Toxicology and Teratology* 8, no. 5 (1986): 509–19.

Lu, Chengsheng, et al. "Organic Diets Significantly Lower Children's Dietary Exposure to Organophosphorus Pesticides." *Environmental Health Perspectives* 114, no. 2 (2006): 260–63.

Lustig, Robert. *Fat Chance: Beating the Odds Against Sugar, Processed Food, Obesity, and Disease.* New York: Hudson Street Press, 2012.

National Academy of Sciences' National Research Council Committee on Cereals. "Cereal Enrichment in Perspective 1958."

Nishimura, R.Y., et al. "Dietary Polyunsaturated Fatty Acid Intake During Late Pregnancy Affects Fatty Acid Composition of Mature Breast Milk." *Nutrition* 30, no. 6 (2014): 685–89.

Olney, J.W. "Excitotoxic Amino Acids and Neuropsychiatric Disorders." *Annual Review of Pharmacology and Toxicology* 30 (1990): 47–71.

O'Mahonya, S.M., et al. "Serotonin, Tryptophan Metabolism and the Brain-Gut-Microbiome Axis." *Behavioural Brain Research* 277 (2015): 32–48.

Peters J.M., et al. "Processed Meats and Risk of Childhood Leukemia (California, USA)." *Cancer Causes and Control* 5, no. 2 (1994): 195–202.

Planck, Nina. *Real Food for Mother and Baby: The Fertility Diet, Eating for Two, and Baby's First Foods.* New York: Bloomsbury, 2009.

Pogoda, J.M., and S. Preston-Martin. "Maternal Cured Meat Consumption During Pregnancy and Risk of Paediatric Brain Tumour in Offspring: Potentially Harmful Levels of Intake." *Public Health Nutrition* 4, no. 2 (2001): 183–89.

Pomara, N., et al. "Excitatory Amino Acid Concentrations in CSF of Patients with Alzheimer's Disease." *Biological Psychiatry* 27, no. 91A (1990).

Preston-Martin, S., et al. "Maternal Consumption of Cured Meats and Vitamins in Relation to Pediatric Brain Tumors." *Cancer Epidemiology, Biomarkers & Prevention* 5, no. 8 (1996): 599–605.

Preston-Martin, et al. "N-Nitroso Compounds and Childhood Brain Tumors: A Case-Control Study." *Cancer Research* 42, no. 12 (1982): 5240–45.

Preston-Martin, S., and W. Lijinsky. "Cured Meats and Childhood Cancer." *Cancer Causes and Control* 5, no. 5 (1994): 484–86.

Public Health Agency of Canada. "Obesity in Canada — Snapshot." Strategic Issues Management Division, Ottawa, 2009. www.phac-aspc.gc.ca.

Renault, T.R., et al. "Fructose, Pregnancy and Later Life Impacts." *Clinical and Experimental Pharmacology and Physiology* 40, no. 11 (2013): 824–37. doi:10.1111/1440-1681.12162.

Sakurai, M. "Sugar-Sweetened Beverage and Diet Soda Consumption and the 7-Year Risk for Type 2 Diabetes Mellitus in Middle-Aged Japanese Men." *European Journal of Nutrition* 53, no. 1 (2014): 251–58. doi:10.1007/s00394-013-0523-9.

Sarasua, S., and D.A. Savitz. "Cured and Broiled Meat Consumption in Relation to Childhood Cancer: Denver, Colorado (United States)." *Cancer Causes and Control* 5, no. 2 (1994): 141–48.

Sauerwein, Kristina. "High-Fructose Diet During Pregnancy May Harm Placenta, Restrict Fetal Growth." Washington University School of Medicine in St. Louis. May 4, 2016. https://medicine.wustl.edu/news/high-fructose-diet-pregnancy-may-harm-placenta-restrict-fetal-growth.

Schernhammer, Eva, et al. "Consumption of Artificial Sweetener and Sugar-Containing Soda and Risk of Lymphoma and Leukemia in Men and Women." *American Journal of Clinical Nutrition* 96, no. 6 (2012): 1419–28. doi:10.3945/ajcn.111.030833.

Simopoulos, A.P. "Evolutionary Aspects of Diet, the Omega-6/Omega-3 Ratio and Genetic Variation: Nutritional Implications for Chronic Diseases." *Biomedicine & Pharmacotherapy* 60, no. 9 (2006): 502–07. doi:10.1016/j.biopha.2006.07.080.

Sloboda, Deborah M. "Early Life Exposure to Fructose and Offspring Phenotype: Implications for Long Term Metabolic Homeostasis." *Journal of Obesity* (2014). doi:10.1155/2014/203474.

Soffritti, Morando, et al. "First Experimental Demonstration of the Multipotential Carcinogenic Effects of Aspartame Administered in the Feed to Sprague-Dawley Rats." *Environmental Health Perspectives* 114, no. 3 (2006): 379–85.

Soffritti, Morando, Fiorella Belpoggi, and Michelina Lauriola. "Life-Span Exposure to Low Doses of Aspartame Beginning During Prenatal Life Increases Cancer Effects in Rats." *Environmental Health Perspectives* 115, no. 9 (2007): 1293–92.

Stevens, L.J., et al. "Mechanisms of Behavioral, Atopic, and Other Reactions to Artificial Food Colors in Children." *Nutrition Reviews* 71, no. 5 (2013): 268–81. doi:10.1111/nure.12023.

Swanson, J.M., S. Entringer, C. Buss, et al. "Developmental Origins of Health and Disease: Environmental Exposures." *Seminars in Reproductive Medicine* 27, no. 5 (2009): 391–402. doi:10.1055/s-0029-1237427.

Thompson, Lilian U. "Potential Health Benefits and Problems Associated with Antinutrients in Foods." *Food Research International* (1993). doi:10.1016/0963-9969(93)90069-U.

Tobacman, J.K. "Review of Harmful Gastrointestinal Effects of Carrageenan in Animal Experiments." *Environmental Health Perspectives* 109, no. 10 (2001): 983–94.

UK Healthy and Safety Executive. The Expert Committee on Pesticide Residues in Food (PRiF). *Annual Report 2012*.

Vighi, G., et al. "Allergy and the Gastrointestinal System." *Clinical and Experimental Immunology* 153, no. 1 (2008): 3–6. doi:10.1111/j.1365-2249.2008.03713.x.

Wadhwa, P.D., et al. "Developmental Origins of Health and Disease: Brief History of the Approach and Current Focus on Epigenetic Mechanisms."

Seminars in Reproductive Medicine: 27, no. 5 (2009): 358–68. doi:10.1055/s-0029-1237424.

Wagner C.L., et al. "Health characteristics and outcomes of NICHD and Thrasher Research Fund (TRF): vitamin D (VITD) supplementation trials during pregnancy," Vitamin D Workshop, presented June, 2012.

Wagner, C.L., et al. "High-Dose Vitamin D3 Supplementation in a Cohort of Breastfeeding Mothers and Their Infants: A 6-Month Follow-up Pilot Study." *Breastfeed Medicine* 1, no. 2 (2006): 59–70.

Willett, W.C., et al. "Intake of Trans Fatty Acids and Risk of Coronary Heart Disease Among Women." *Lancet* 341, no. 8845 (1993): 581–85.

Winchester, Paul D., Jordan Huskins, and Jun Ying. "Agrichemicals in Surface Water and Birth Defects in the United States." *Acta Paediatrica* 98, no. 4 (2009): 664–69. doi:10.1111/j.1651-2227.2008.01207.x.

Young, Emma. "Gut Instincts: The Secrets of Your Second Brain." *New Scientist*, December 18, 2012.

Chapter 3: Greening the Growing Fetus and The Natural Pregnancy Handbook

Andra, S.S., C. Austin, and M. Arora. "The Tooth Exposome in Children's Health Research." *Current Opinion in Pediatrics* 28, no. 2 (2016): 221–27. doi:10.1097/MOP.0000000000000327.

Bajwa, U., and K.S. Sandhu. "Effect of Handling and Processing on Pesticide Residues in Food: A Review." *Journal of Food Science and Technology* 51, no. 2 (2014): 201–20. doi:10.1007/s13197-011-0499-5.

Bellinger, D.C. "A Strategy for Comparing the Contributions of Environmental Chemicals and Other Risk Factors to Neurodevelopment of Children." *Environmental Health Perspectives* 120, no. 4 (2012): 501–07. doi:10.1289/ehp.1104170.

Bethel, C., et al. "A National and State Profile of Leading Health Problems and Health Care Quality for U.S. Children." *Academic Pediatrics* 11, no. 3 (2011): S22–33. doi:10.1016/j.acap.2010.08.011.

Bilbrey, Jenna. "BPA-Free Plastic Containers May Be Just as Hazardous," *Scientific American*, August 11, 2014.

Blanding, Michael, and Madeline Drexler. "The E-Cig Quandary." *Harvard Public Health*, November 2016. www.hsph.harvard.edu/magazine/magazine_article/the-e-cig-quandary.

Bose-O'Reilly, S., et al. "Mercury Exposure and Children's Health." *Current Problems in Pediatric and Adolescent Health Care* 40, no. 8 (2010): 186–215. doi:10.1016/j.cppeds.2010.07.002.

Carnansky, Rachel. "What Toxins Have You Been Exposed To? Your Baby Teeth May Hold the Answer." *Washington Post*, July 11, 2016.

Charness, Michael E., et al. "Drinking During Pregnancy and the Developing Brain: Is Any Amount Safe?" *Trends in Cognitive Sciences* 20, no. 2 (2016): 80–82.

Curry, Andrew. "Exploring Why Gestational Diabetes Leads to Type 2: Harvard Researcher Frank Hu Taps Important Diabetes and Pregnancy Data." *Diabetes Forecast: The Healthy Living Magazine*, January 2015. www.diabetesforecast.org/2015/jan-feb/exploring-gestational-diabetes-leads-type-2.html. Accessed November 29, 2016.

Federation of American Societies for Experimental Biology. "Low Dose Of Caffeine When Pregnant May Damage Heart of Offspring for a Lifetime." *ScienceDaily*. www.sciencedaily.com/releases/2008/12/081216133440.htm. Accessed November 8, 2016.

Forestier, F., et al. "The Passage of Fluoride Across the Placenta: An Intra-uterine Study." *Journal de Gynécologie Obstétrique et Biologie de la Reproduction (Paris)* 19, no. 2 (1990): 171–75.

Grandjean, P., et al. "Cognitive Deficit in 7-Year-Old Children with Prenatal Exposure to Methlymerucry." *Neurotoxicology Teratology* 19, no. 6 (1997): 417–28.

Gregory, Andrew. "Pregnant Women Warned 'E-Cigarettes Could Harm Your Unborn Baby and Are as Bad as Tobacco.'" *Mirror*, February 11, 2016.

Hicks, Monique B., Y-H. Peggy Hsieh, and Leonard N. Bell. "Tea Preparation and Its Influence on Methylxanthine Concentration." *Food Research International* 29, nos. 3–4 (1996): 325–30.

Jefferson, W.N., H.B. Patisaul, and C.J. Williams. "Reproductive Consequences of Developmental Phytoestrogen Exposure." *Reproduction (Cambridge, England)* 143, no. 3 (2012): 247–60. doi:10.1530/REP-11-0369.

Karagas, M.R. "Evidence on the Human Health Effects of Low-Level Methyl Mercury Exposure." *Environmental Health Perspectives* 120, no. 6 (2012): 799–806.

Kennedy, Robert F., Jr. *Thimerosal: Let the Science Speak*. New York: Skyhorse, 2014.

Knopik, V.S., M.A. Maccani, S. Francazio, et al. "The Epigenetics of Maternal Cigarette Smoking During Pregnancy and Effects on Child Development." *Development and Psychopathology* 24, no. 4 (2012): 1377–90. doi:10.1017/S0954579412000776.

Lanphear, Bruce. "The Impact of Toxins on the Developing Brain." *Annual Review of Public Health* 36 (2015): 211–30. doi:10.1146/annurev-publhealth-031912-114413.

Li, X.S., J.L. Zhi, and R.O. Gao. "Effect of Fluoride Exposure on Intelligence in Children." *Fluoride* 28, no. 4 (1995): 189–92.

Liew, Z., et al. "Acetaminophen Use During Pregnancy, Behavioral Problems, and Hyperkinetic Disorders." *JAMA Pediatrics* 168, no. 4 (2014): 313–20.

Miller, A.R. "Diagnostic Nomenclature for Foetal Alcohol Spectrum Disorders: The Continuing Challenge of Causality." *Child: Care, Health and Development* 39, no. 6 (2013): 810–15. doi:10.1111/cch.12017.

Miller, M.W., et al. "Hyperthermic Teratogenicity, Thermal Dose and Diagnostic Ultrasound During Pregnancy: Implications of New Standards on Tissue Heating." *International Journal of Hyperthermia* 18, no. 5 (2002): 361–84.

Moore, Charles W. "Mercury Fillings: A Time Bomb in Your Head." *Natural Life Magazine*. www.life.ca/naturallife/9702/mercury.htm. Accessed November 14, 2016.

Morrel, Sally Fallon, and Thomas Cowan. *The Nourishing Traditions Book of Baby & Childcare*. Washington, DC: New Trends, 2013.

Mutter, J., et al. "Amalgam Studies: Disregarding Basic Principles of Mercury Toxicity." *International Journal of Hygiene and Environmental Health* 207, no. 4 (2004): 391–97.

Nezvalová-Henriksen, K., O. Spigset, and H. Nordeng. "Effects of Ibuprofen, Diclofenac, Naproxen, and Piroxicam on the Course of Pregnancy and Pregnancy Outcome: A Prospective Cohort Study." *BJOG* 120, no. 8 (2013): 948–59.

Peedikayil, F.C., P. Sreenivasan, and A. Narayanan. "Effect of Coconut Oil in Plaque-Related Gingivitis: A Preliminary Report." *Nigerian Medical Journal: Journal of the Nigeria Medical Association* 56, no. 2 (2015): 143–47. doi:10.4103/0300-1652.153406.

Peritz, Ingrid. "Canadian Doctor Averted Disaster by Keeping Thalidomide out of the U.S." *Globe and Mail*, November 24, 2014.

Pesticide Action Network. "Reducing Hazardous Pesticide Practice in Coffee Supply Chains." July 2008. www.pan-uk.org/attachments/318_f&f-coffee.pdf.

Planck, Nina. *Real Food for Mother and Baby: The Fertility Diet, Eating for Two, and Baby's First Foods*. New York: Bloomsbury, 2009.

Raffelock, Dean, Robert Rountree, and Virginia Hopkins. *A Natural Guide to Pregnancy and Postpartum Health: The First Book by Doctors that Really Addresses Pregnancy Recovery*. New York: Penguin Putnam, 2002.

Rudge, C.V., et al. "The Placenta as a Barrier for Toxic and Essential Elements in Paired Maternal and Cord Blood Samples of South African Delivering Women." *Journal of Environmental Monitoring* 11, no. 7 (2009): 1322–30. doi:10.1039/b903805a.

Samuel, Eugenie. "Fetuses Can Hear Ultrasound Examinations." *New Scientist*, December 4, 2001. www.newscientist.com/article/dn1639-fetuses-can-hear-ultrasound-examinations-.html. Accessed May 11, 2006.

Selevan, S.G., C.A. Kimmel, and P. Mendola. "Identifying Critical Windows of Exposure for Children's Health." *Environmental Health Perspectives* 108, Suppl. 3 (2000): 451–55.

Shrim, A., et al. "Pregnancy Outcome Following Use of Large Doses of Vitamin B6 in the First Trimester." *Journal of Obstetrics and Gynaecology* 26, no. 8 (2006): 749–51.

Society of Obstetricians and Gynaecologists of Canada. "Ultrasound in Pregnancy." http://pregnancy.sogc.org/routine-tests/ultrasound-in-pregnancy. Accessed November 30, 2016.

Spittle, B., et al. "Intelligence and Fluoride Exposure in New Zealand Children (Abstract)." *Fluoride* 31, no. 13 (1998).

Tam, C., A. Erebara, and A. Einarson. "Food-Borne Illnesses During Pregnancy: Prevention and Treatment." *Canadian Family Physician* 56, no. 4 (2010): 341–43.

Thalidomide Victims Association of Canada. "Thalidomide: The Canadian Tragedy." www.thalidomide.ca/the-canadian-tragedy.

Tobias, D.K., et al. "Healthful Dietary Patterns and Type 2 Diabetes Risk Among Women with a History of Gestational Diabetes." *Archives of Internal Medicine* 172, no. 20 (2012): 1566–72. doi:10.1001/archinternmed.2012.3747.

United States Environmental Protection Agency. "Persistent Organic Pollutants: A Global Issue, A Global Response." www.epa.gov/international-cooperation/persistent-organic-pollutants-global-issue-global-response.

United States Food and Drug Administration, "For Consumers: Seven Things Pregnant Women and Parents Need to Know About Arsenic in Rice and Rice Cereal" *Consumer Health Information*. www.fda.gov/downloads/ForConsumers/ConsumerUpdates/UCM493757.pdf. Accessed November 14, 2016.

University of Gothenburg. "Coffee and Tea During Pregnancy Affect Fetal Growth." *ScienceDaily*, March 11, 2013. www.sciencedaily.com/releases/2013/03/130311101649.htm.

Warren, J.L. "Bayesian Multinomial Probit Modeling of Daily Windows of Susceptibility for Maternal PM2.5 Exposure and Congenital Heart Defects." *Statistics in Medicine* 35, no. 16 (2016): 2786–801. doi:10.1002/sim.6891.

Wendler, Christopher C., et al. "Embryonic Caffeine Exposure Induces Adverse Effects in Adulthood." *FASEB Journal* 23, no. 4 (2009) doi:10.1096/fj.08-124941.

Weng, X., R. Odouli, and D.K. Li. "Maternal Caffeine Consumption During Pregnancy and the Risk of Miscarriage: A Prospective Cohort Study." *American Journal of Obstetrics and Gynecology* 198, no. 3 (2008): 279.

Woodruff, T.J., A.R. Zota, and J.M. Schwartz. "Environmental Chemicals in Pregnant Women in the United States: NHANES 2003–2004." *Environmental Health Perspectives* 119, no. 6 (2011): 878–85.

Wu, Haotian, et al. "Environmental Susceptibility of the Sperm Epigenome During Windows of Male Germ Cell Development." *Current Environmental Health Reports* 2, no. 4 (2015): 356–66. doi:10.1007/s40572-015-0067-7.

Yang, C.Z., et al. "Most Plastic Products Release Estrogenic Chemicals: A Potential Health Problem That Can Be Solved." *Environmental Health Perspectives* 119, no. 7 (2011): 989–96. doi:10.1289/ehp.1003220.

Yang, Y., et al. "The Effects of High Levels of Fluoride and Iodine on Intellectual Ability and the Metabolism of Fluoride and Iodine." *Chinese Journal of Epidemiology* 15, no. 4 (1994): 296–98.

Chapter 4: Greening Your Home and The Green Baby Shower Handbook

Baiz, Nour, et al. "Maternal Exposure to Air Pollution Before and During Pregnancy Related to Changes in Newborn's Cord Blood Lymphocyte Xubpopulations: The EDEN Study Cohort." *BMC Pregnancy Childbirth* 11, no. 87 (2011). doi:10.1186/1471-2393-11-87.

Bellieni, C.V., et al. "Exposure to Electromagnetic Fields from Laptop Use of 'Laptop' Computers." *Archives of Environmental and Occupational Health* 67, no. 1 (2012): 31–36. doi:10.1080/19338244.2011.564232.

Cech, R., N. Leitgeb, and M. Pediaditis. "Current Densities in a Pregnant Woman Model Induced by Simultaneous ELF Electric and Magnetic Field Exposure." *Physics in Medicine and Biology* 53, no. 1 (2008): 177–86. doi:10.1088/0031-9155/53/1/012.

Chen, A., et al. "Prenatal Polybrominated Diphenyl Ether Exposures and Neurodevelopment in U.S. Children Through 5 Years of Age: The HOME Study." *Environmental Health Perspectives* 122, no. 8 (2014): 856–62. doi:10.1289/ehp.1307562.

Cunnington, D., M.F. Junge, and A.T. Fernando. "Insomnia: Prevalence, Consequences and Effective Treatment." *Medical Journal of Australia* 199, no. 8 (2013): S36–40.

DefenderShield. "EMF Exposure During Pregnancy Increases Risk of Asthma in Children." www.defendershield.com/emf-exposure-pregnancy-increases-risk-asthma-children.

Figà-Talamanca, I., P. Nardone, and C. Giliberti. "Exposure to Electromagnetic Fields and Human Reproduction: The Epidemiologic Evidence." In "Non-thermal Effects and Mechanisms of Interaction Between Electromagnetic Fields and Living Matter." *European Journal of Oncology – Library* 5 (2010): 387–402.

Franck, U., et al. "Prenatal VOC Exposure and Redecoration Are Related to Wheezing in Early Infancy." *Environment International* 73 (2014): 393–401. doi:10.1016/j.envint.2014.08.013.

Gibson, Rachel, and Travis Madsen. "Toxic Baby Furniture: The Latest Case for Making Products Safe from the Start." *Environment California Research and Policy Center*, May 2008.

Hansen, C.A., A.G. Barnett, and G. Pritchard. "The Effect of Ambient Air Pollution During Early Pregnancy on Fetal Ultrasonic Measurements During Mid-Pregnancy." *Environmental Health Perspectives* 116, no. 3 (2008): 362–69. doi:10.1289/ehp.10720.

Jing, J., et al. "The Influence of Microwave Radiation from Cellular Phone on Fetal Rat Brain." *Electromagnetic Biology and Medicine* 31, no. 1 (2012): 57–66. doi:10.3109/15368378.2011.624652.

John Hopkins University. "Study: Even a Little Air Pollution May Have Long-Term Health Effects on Developing Fetus." April 27, 2016. www.jhsph. edu/news/news-releases/2016/study-even-a-little-air-pollution-may-have-long-term-health-effects-on-developing-fetus.html.

Kane, R.C. "A Possible Association Between Fetal/Neonatal Exposure to Radiofrequency Electromagnetic Radiation and the Increased Incidence of Autism Spectrum Disorders (ASD)." *Medical Hypotheses* 62, no. 2 (2004): 195–97.

Khoudja, R.Y., et al. "Better IVF Outcomes Following Improvements in Laboratory Air Quality." *Journal of Assisted Reproduction and Genetics* 30, no. 1 (2013): 69–76. doi:10.1007/s10815-012-9900-1.

Kim, Sung, Rolf U. Halden, and Timothy J. Buckley. "Volatile Organic Compounds in Human Milk: Method and Measurements." *Environmental Science and Technology* 41, no. 5 (2007): 1662–67. doi:10.1021/es062362y.

Li, D., H. Chen, and R. Odouli. "Maternal Exposure to Magnetic Fields During Pregnancy in Relation to the Risk of Asthma in Offspring." *Archives of Pediatric and Adolescent Medicine* 165, no. 10 (2011): 945–50. doi:10.1001/archpediatrics.2011.135.

Maroziene, Ligita, and Regina Grazuleviciene. "Maternal Exposure to Low-Level Air Pollution and Pregnancy Outcomes: A Population-Based Study." *Environmental Health* 1, no. 1 (2002): 6. doi: 10.1186/1476-069X-1-6.

McGwin, Gerald, Jeffrey Lienert, and John I. Kennedy Jr. "Formaldehyde Exposure and Asthma in Children: A Systematic Review." *Environmental Health Perspectives* 118, no. 3 (2010): 313–17.

Park, Alice. "How Air Pollution Affects Babies in the Womb." *Time*, March 25, 2015.

Peterson, Bradley, et al. "Effects of Prenatal Exposure to Air Pollutants

(Polycyclic Aromatic Hydrocarbons) on the Development of Brain White Matter, Cognition, and Behavior in Later Childhood." *JAMA Psychiatry* 72, no. 6 (2015): 531–40. doi:10.1001/jamapsychiatry.2015.57.

Sherriff, A., et al. "Frequent Use of Chemical Household Products Is Associated with Persistent Wheezing in Pre-school Age Children." *Thorax* 60, no. 1 (2005): 45–49.

Šrám, Radim J., et al. "Ambient Air Pollution and Pregnancy Outcomes: A Review of the Literature." *Environmental Health Perspectives* 113, no. 4 (2005): 375–82. doi:10.1289/ehp.6362.

Woodruff, T., et al. "Disparities in Exposure to Air Pollution During Pregnancy." *Environmental Health Perspectives* 111, no. 7 (2003): 942–46.

Chapter 5: Greening Your Beauty Care and The DIY Green Beauty Care Handbook

Advanced Science News Staff. "Fetal Risk of Nanoparticle Exposure Assessed." *Advanced Science News*, November 26, 2012. www.advancedsciencenews.com/fetal-risk-of-nanoparticle-exposure-assessed.

Aiello, Allison, Elaine L. Larson, and Stuart B. Levy. "Consumer Antibacterial Soaps: Effective or Just Risky?" *Clinical Infectious Diseases* 45, no. 2 (2007): S137–S147. doi:10.1086/519255.

Arthur, B. and R. Stein. "Exploring the Invisible Universe That Lives on Us — and in Us." *NPR*, November 4, 2013. www.npr.org/sections/health-shots/2013/11/01/242361826/exploring-the-invisible-universe-that-lives-on-us-and-in-us. Accessed February 23, 2014.

Cimitile, Matthew. "Nanoparticles from Sunscreen Damage Microbes." *Environmental Health News*, March 24, 2009.

Cook, Linda S., Mary L. Kamb, and Noel S. Weiss. "Perineal Powder Exposure and the Risk of Ovarian Cancer." *American Journal of Epidemiology* 145, no. 5 (1997): 459–65.

Darbre, P.D. "Aluminium, Antiperspirants and Breast Cancer." *Journal of Inorganic Biochemistry* 99, no. 9 (2005): 1912–19.

Deacon, Gillian. *There's Lead in Your Lipstick*. Toronto: Penguin Group Canada, 2010.

Environment and Climate Change Canada. "Microbeads — A Science Summary," July, 2015. Accessed online at https://www.ec.gc.ca/ese-ees/default.asp?lang=En&n=ADDA4C5F-1.

Fitzgerald, Kara. "Your Skin Microbiome: Why It's Essential for a Healthy Glow." *MindBodyGreen*, March 8, 2016.

Gertig, Dorota M., et al. "Prospective Study of Talc Use and Ovarian Cancer."

Journal of the National Cancer Institute 92, no. 3 (2000): 249–52.

Harvey, P.W. "Parabens, Oestrogenicity, Underarm Cosmetics and Breast Cancer: A Perspective on a Hypothesis." *Journal of Applied Toxicology* 23, no. 5 (2003): 285–88.

Health Canada. "Guidance on Heavy Metal Impurities in Cosmetics." July 2012. www.hc-sc.gc.ca/cps-spc/pubs/indust/heavy_metals-metaux_lourds/index-eng.php.

Hong, S., et al. "Association Between Exposure to Antimicrobial Household Products and Allergic Symptoms." *Environmenal Health and Toxicology* 29 (2014). doi:10.5620/eht.e2014017.

Kawahara, M., and M. Kato-Negishi. "Link Between Aluminum and the Pathogenesis of Alzheimer's Disease: The Integration of the Aluminum and Amyloid Cascade Hypotheses." *International Journal of Alzheimer's Disease* (2011). doi:10.4061/2011/276393.

Keelan, Jeffrey. "Nanotoxicology: Nanoparticles versus the Placenta." *Nature Nanotechnology* 6, no. 5 (2011): 263–64. doi:10.1038/nnano.2011.65.

Morris, Robert D. "Chlorination, Chlorination By-products, and Cancer: A Meta-analysis." *American Journal of Public Health* 82, no. 7 (1992): 955–63.

National Association for Holistic Aromatherapy. "Exploring Aromatherapy: Pregnancy Safety." http://naha.org/explore-aromatherapy/safety/#pregnancy. Accessed December 30, 2016.

Rice, Maureen. "Revealed: The 515 Chemicals Women Put on Their Bodies Every Day." *Daily Mail*, November 20, 2009. www.dailymail.co.uk/femail/beauty/article-1229275/Revealed--515-chemicals-women-bodies-day.html.

Schmidt, C.W. "Uncertain Inheritance: Transgenerational Effects of Environmental Exposures." *Environmental Health Perspectives* 121, no. 10 (2013): A298–A303. doi:10.1289/ ehp.121-A298.

Seltenrich, Nate. "New Link in the Food Chain? Marine Plastic Pollution and Seafood Safety." *Environmental Health Perspectives* 123, no. 2 (2015): A34–A41. doi:10.1289/ehp.123-A34.

Sepmag. "Microbeads/Nanoparticles for Cell Sorting." November 13, 2014. www.sepmag.eu/blog/bid/398786/Microbeads-Nanoparticles-for-Cell-Sorting. Accessed December 10, 2016.

Silverman, Jacob. "Why Is the World's Biggest Landfill in the Pacific Ocean?" *How Stuff Works*, September 19, 2007. http://science.howstuffworks.com/environmental/earth/oceanography/great-pacific-garbage-patch.htm. Accessed December 10, 2016.

Steinberg, David C. "Regulatory Review – US and Canada Updates: Canadian Cosmetic Harmonization and the FDA's Claim Crackdown." *Cosmetics and Toiletries* 128, no. 1 (2013): 20–27.

Titus-Ernstoff, et al. "Birth Defects in the Sons and Daughters of Women Who Were Exposed In Utero to Diethylstilbestrol (DES)." *International*

Journal of Andrology 33, no. 2 (2009): 377–84. doi:10.1111/j.1365-2605.2009.01010.x.

Umezawa, M., et al. "Effect of Fetal Exposure to Titanium Dioxide Nanoparticle on Brain Development — Brain Region Information." *The Journal of Toxicological Sciences* 37, no. 6 (2012): 1247–52.

Urban, J., et al. "The Effect of Habitual and Experimental Antiperspirant and Deodorant Product Use on the Armpit Microbiome." *PeerJ* 4 (2016). doi:10.7717/peerj.1605.

Verbeeck, R.M., F.C. Driessens, and J. Rotgans. "The Use of Aluminum-Containing Toothpaste and Its Potential Risk." *Revue Belge de Medecine Dentaire (1984)* 45, no. 2 (1990): 53–58; discussion 58–59.

Zeh, Jeanne A., et al. "From Father to Son: Transgenerational Effect of Tetracycline on Sperm Viability." *Scientific Reports* 2, no. 375 (2012). doi:10.1038/srep00375.

Chapter 6: Greening Birth, Breastfeeding, and Beyond; and Chapter 7: Greening the Fourth Trimester and Preparing for Postpartum Bliss

American Academy of Pediatrics. "Breastfeeding and the Use of Human Milk." *Pediatrics* 115, no. 2 (2005): 496–506.

Ball, T.M., and A.L. Wright. "Health Care Costs of Formula-Feeding in the First Year of Life." *Pediatrics* 103, no. 4.2 (1999): 870–76.

Belfort, Mandy B., Sheryl Rifas-Shiman, Ken Kleinman, et al. "Infant Feeding and Childhood Cognition at Ages 3 and 7 Years: Effects of Breastfeeding Duration and Exclusivity." *JAMA Pediatrics* 167, no. 9 (2013): 836–44. doi:10.1001/jamapediatrics.2013.455.

Benoit, C., C. Stengel, R. Phillips, et al. "Privatisation and Marketisation of Post-birth Care: The Hidden Costs for New Mothers." *International Journal for Equity in Health* 11, no. 62 (2012). doi:10.1186/1475-9276-11-61.

Bonyata, K. "Q & A: Preventing Thrush." *KellyMom*, 2011. http://kellymom.com/bf/concerns/child/preventing-thrush. Accessed March 7, 2015.

British Columbia Perinatal Health Program. *Caesarean Birth Task Force Report 2008.*

Brizendine, Louann. *The Female Brain.* New York: Harmony Books, 2007.

Cabrera-Rubio, Raul, et al. "The Human Milk Microbiome Changes Over Lactation and Is Shaped by Maternal Weight and Mode of Delivery," *American Journal of Clinical Nutrition* 96, no. 3 (2012): 544–51. doi:10.3945/ajcn.112.037382.

Canadian Paediatric Society Nutrition and Gastroenterology Committee. "Exclusive Breastfeeding Should Continue to Six Months." *Paediatrics & Child Health* 10, no. 3 (2005): 148.

Collaborative Group on Hormonal Factors in Breast Cancer. "Breast Cancer and Breastfeeding: Collaborative Reanalysis of Individual Data from 47 Epidemiological Studies in 30 Countries, Including 50,302 Women with Breast Cancer and 96,973 Women without the Disease." *Lancet* 360, no. 9328 (2002): 187–95. doi:10.1016/S0140-6736(02)09454-0.

Dekker, Rebecca. "Evidence for the Vitamin K Shot in Newborns." *Evidence Based Birth*, March 18, 2014. https://evidencebasedbirth.com/evidence-for-the-vitamin-k-shot-in-newborns.

Dominguez-Bello, Maria G., et al. "Delivery Mode Shapes the Acquisition and Structure of the Initial Microbiota Across Multiple Body Habitats in Newborns." *Proceedings of the National Academy of Sciences* 107, no. 26 (2010): 11971–975.

Dominguez-Bello, Maria G., et al. "Partial Restoration of the Microbiota of Cesarean-Born Infants via Vaginal Microbial Transfer." *Nature Medicine* 22, no. 3 (2016): 250–53. doi:10.1038/nm.4039.

Gill, Sara L., Elizabeth Reifsnider, and Joseph Lucke. "Effects of Support on the Initiation and Duration of Breastfeeding." *Western Journal of Nursing Research* 29, no. 6 (2007): 708–23.

Gryder, Laura, et al. "Effects of Human Maternal Placentophagy on Maternal Postpartum Iron Status: A Randomized, Double Blind, Placebo Controlled Pilot Study." *Journal of Midwifery and Women's Health* 62, no. 1 (2016): 68–79. doi:10.1111/jmwh.12549.

Hall, Harriet. "Circumcision: What Does Science Say?" *Science-Based Medicine*, November 4, 2008. https://sciencebasedmedicine.org/circumcision-what-does-science-say. Accessed December 7, 2016.

Harder, T., et al. "Duration of Breastfeeding and Risk of Overweight: A Meta-analysis." *American Journal of Epidemiology* 162, no. 5 (2005):397–403.

Health Canada. "Nutrition for Healthy Term Infants – Statement of the Joint Working Group: Canadian Paediatric Society, Dieticians of Canada and Health Canada. Breastfeeding." www.hc-sc.gc.ca/fn-an/pubs/infant-nourrisson/nut_infant_nourrisson_term_3-eng.php.

Hospital for Sick Children. "Breastfeeding and Drugs." www.motherisk.org/women/breastfeeding.jsp.

Jiménez, E., et al. "Oral Administration of Lactobacillus Strains Isolated from Breast Milk as an Alternative for the Treatment of Infectious Mastitis During Lactation." *Applied and Environmental Microbiology* 74, no. 15 (2008): 4650–55.

Kim, P., et al. "The Plasticity of Human Maternal Brain: Longitudinal Changes in Brain Anatomy During the Early Postpartum Period." *Behavioral*

Neuroscience 124, no. 5 (2010): 695–700. doi:10.1037/a0020884.

Leeb, Kira, et al. "Are There Socio-Economic Differences in Caesarean Section Rates in Canada?" *Healthcare Policy* 1, no. 1 (2005): 48–54.

Phillips, Raylene. "The Sacred Hour: Uninterrupted Skin-to-Skin Contact Immediately After Birth." *Newborn and Infant Nursing Reviews* 13, no. 2 (2013): 67–72.

Quinn, E.A. (2014). "Human Milk Has a Microbiome – and the Bacteria Are Protecting Mothers and Infants!" *Biomarkers & Milk*, December 14, 2014. http://biomarkersandmilk.blogspot.ca/2014/12/human-milk-has-microbiome-and-bacteria.html. Accessed February 23, 2014.

Reardon, S. "Babies' Weak Immune Systems Let Good Bacteria In." *Nature*, November 6, www.nature.com/news/babies-weak-immune-systems-let-good-bacteria-in-1.14112. Accessed February 23, 2014.

Rettner, R. "Probiotics May Help Prevent Infant Gut Disorders." *Live Science*, January 13, 2014. www.livescience.com/42538-probiotics-infant-gut-disorders-colic.html. Accessed February 23, 2014.

Rogier, E.W., et al. "Secretory Antibodies in Breast Milk Promote Long-Term Intestinal Homeostasis by Regulating the Gut Microbiota and Host Gene Expression." *Proceedings of the National Academy of Sciences* 111, no. 8 (2014): 3074–79.

Rush, J., et al. "The Effects of Whirlpool Baths in Labor: A Randomized, Controlled Trial." *Birth: Issues in Perinatal Care* 23, no. 3 (1996): 136–43.

Selander, Jodi, et al. "Human Maternal Placentophagy: A Survey of Self-Reported Motivations and Experiences Associated with Placenta Consumption." *Ecology of Food and Nutrition* 52, no. 2 (2013): 93–115.

Shearer, M.J. "Vitamin K Deficiency Bleeding (VKDB) in Early Infancy." *Blood Reviews* 23, no. 2 (2009): 49–59.

Smith, Anne. "When Breastfeeding Doesn't Work Out," *Breastfeeding Basics.* September, 2016. www.breastfeedingbasics.com/articles/when-breastfeeding-doesnt-work-out.

Soykova-Pachnerova, E., et al. "Placenta as a Lactagogon," *Gynaecologia* 138, no. 6: 617–27.

Stanford University. "Effects of Oral Probiotic Supplementation on Group B Strep (GBS) Rectovaginal Colonization in Pregnancy." ClinicalTrials.gov: NCT01479478. Approved October 2016.

Thanabalasuriar, Ajitha, and Paul Kubes. "Neonates, Antibiotics and the Microbiome." *Nature Medicine* 20, no. 5 (2014): 469–70. doi:10.1038/nm.3558.

Vallaeys, Charlotte. "Replacing Mother: Imitating Human Breast Milk in the Laboratory." *Cornucopia Institute*, January 2008.

Women's Health Data Resource. www.womenshealthdata.ca. Accessed December 1, 2016.

World Health Organization. "Trends in Maternal Mortality: 1990 to 2015 Estimates by WHO, UNICEF, UNFPA, World Bank Group and the United Nations Population Division Executive Summary." 2015.

Yong, E. "How Breast Milk Engineers a Baby's Gut (and Gut Microbes)." *National Geographic*, February 3, 2014. http://phenomena. nationalgeographic.com/2014/02/03/how-breast-milk-engineers-a-babys-gut-and-gut-microbes.

Chapter 8: Greening for Your Future Fertility

Adebamowo, Clement A., et al. "High School Dietary Dairy Intake and Teenage Acne." *Journal of the American Academy of Dermatology* 52, no. 2 (2005): 207–14. doi:10.1016/j.jaad.2004.08.007.

Afeiche, M., et al. "Dairy Food Intake in Relation to Semen Quality and Reproductive Hormone Levels among Physically Active Young Men." *Human Reproduction (Oxford, England)* 28, no. 8 (2013): 2265–75.

Andersen, A.M.N., et al. "Advanced Paternal Age and Risk of Fetal Death: A Cohort Study." *American Journal of Epidemiology* 160, no. 12 (2004): 1214–22. doi:10.1093/aje/kwh332.

Anderson, L.M., et al. "Preconceptional Fasting of Fathers Alters Serum Glucose in Offspring of Mice." *Nutrition* 22, no. 3 (2006): 327–31.

Barrett, J.R. "The Science of Soy: What Do We Really Know?" *Environmental Health Perspectives.* 114, no. 6 (2006): A352–A358.

Bolúmar, F., J. Olsen, M. Rebagliato, et al. "Caffeine Intake and Delayed Conception: A European Multicenter Study on Infertility and Subfecundity." European Study Group on Infertility Subfecundity. *American Journal of Epidemiology* 145, no. 4 (1997): 324–34.

Chavarro, Jorge E., et al. "Dietary Fatty Acid Intakes and the Risk of Ovulatory Infertility." *American Journal of Clinical Nutrition* 85, no. 1 (2007): 231–37.

Chavarro, Jorge E., et al. "Soy Food and Isoflavone Intake in Relation to Semen Quality Parameters Among Men from an Infertility Clinic." *Human Reproduction* 23, no. 11 (2008): 2584–90. doi:10.1093/humrep/den243.

Chavarro, Jorge E., et al. "Soy Intake Modifies the Relation Between Urinary Bisphenol A Concentrations and Pregnancy Outcomes Among Women Undergoing Assisted Reproduction." *Journal of Clinical Endocrinology and Metabolism* 101, no. 3 (2016): 1082–90. doi:10.1210/jc.2015-3473.

Chavarro, Jorge E., et al. "Trans Fatty Acid Levels in Sperm Are Associated with Sperm Concentration Among Men from an Infertility Clinic."

Fertility and Sterility 95, no. 5 (2011): 1794–97. doi:10.1016/j.
fertnstert.2010.10.039.

Cheslack-Postava, Keely, Kayuet Liu, and Peter S. Bearman. "Closely Spaced
Pregnancies Are Associated with Increased Odds of Autism in California
Sibling Births." *Pediatrics* 127, no. 2 (2011): 246–53.

Cole, William. "11 Everyday Toxins That Are Harming Your Thyroid."
MindBodyGreen, January 21, 2014. www.mindbodygreen.com/0-
12346/11-everyday-toxins-that-are-harming-your-thyroid.html. Accessed
December 4, 2016.

Conrad, S., et al. "Soy Formula Complicates Management of Congenital
Hypothyroidism." *Archives of Disease in Childhood* 89, no. 1 (2004): 37–40.

Daniel, Kaayla T. *The Whole Soy Story: The Dark Side of America's Favorite
Health Food*. Washington, DC: New Trends, 2005.

Eckert, Linda O., et al. "Relationship of Vaginal Bacteria and Inflammation with
Conception and Early Pregnancy Loss Following In-Vitro Fertilization."
Infectious Diseases in Obstetrics and Gynecology 11, no. 1 (2003): 11–17.

Gillerman, K., N. Rehman, M. Dilgil, et al. "The Impact of Acupuncture
on IVF Success Rates: A Randomised Controlled Trial." Homerton
University Hospital, Homerton Fertility Centre, London, UK, presented
at the European Society of Human Reproduction and Embryology 32nd
Annual Meeting, Helsinki, Finland, July 3–6, 2016.

Gritz, Emily C., and Vineet Bhandari. "The Human Neonatal Gut
Microbiome: A Brief Review." *Frontiers in Pediatrics* 3 (2015): 17.
doi:10.3389/fped.2015.00017.

Harvard Medical School. "Blue Light Has a Dark Side: Exposure to Blue
Light at Night, Emitted by Electronics and Energy-Efficient Lightbulbs,
Harmful to Your Health." *Harvard Health Publications*. Updated
September 2, 2015. Originally published May 2012.

Harvard Medical School. "Our Microbes, Ourselves: Billions of Bacteria Within,
Essential for Immune Function, Are Ours Alone." *ScienceDaily*, June 21,
2012. www.sciencedaily.com/releases/2012/06/120621130643.htm.
Accessed September 26, 2016.

Hatch, E.E., and M.B. Bracken. "Association of Delayed Conception with
Caffeine Consumption." *American Journal of Epidemiology* 138, no. 12
(1993): 1082–92.

Holford, Patrick. *Optimum Nutrition for the Mind*. London: Little Brown
Book Group, 2007.

Hultman, C.M., S. Sandin, S.Z. Levine, et al. "Advancing Paternal Age and
Risk of Autism: New Evidence from a Population-Based Study and a Meta-
analysis of Epidemiological Studies." *Molecular Psychiatry* 16, no. 12 (2011):
1203–12. doi:10.1038/mp.2010.121.

Jensen, T.K. "High Dietary Intake of Saturated Fat Is Associated with Reduced Semen Quality Among 701 Young Danish Men from the General Population." *American Journal of Clinical Nutrition* 97, no. 2 (2013): 411–18. doi:10.3945/ajcn.112.042432.

Langer, Stephen. *Solved: The Riddle of Illness*. New Canaan, CT: Keats, 2000.

Ma, B., L.J. Forney, and J. Ravel. "The Vaginal Microbiome: Rethinking Health and Diseases." *Annual Review of Microbiology* 66 (2012): 371–89. doi:10.1146/annurev-micro-092611-150157.

Mayo Clinic. "Family Planning: Get the Facts About Pregnancy Spacing." www.mayoclinic.org/healthy-lifestyle/getting-pregnant/in-depth/family-planning/art-20044072.

Mendiola, J., et al. "Food Intake and Its Relationship with Semen Quality: A Case-Control Study." *Fertility and Sterility* 91, no. 3 (2009): 812–18. doi:10.1016/j.fertnstert.2008.01.020.

Nierenberg, Cari. "Stay Up Late? How It Could Hurt Your Fertility." *LiveScience*, July 15, 2014. www.livescience.com/46807-night-light-melatonin-fertility-pregnancy.html. Accessed October 4, 2016.

North, K. and J. Golding. "A Maternal Vegetarian Diet in Pregnancy Is Associated with Hypospadias." The ALSPAC Study Team. Avon Longitudinal Study of Pregnancy and Childhood. *BJU International* 85, no. 1 (2000): 107–13.

Pentland, Spence. *Being Fertile: 10 Steps to Help You Overcome the Struggles of Infertility, Get Pregnant, and Create a Happy, Healthy Family*. Vancouver: Yinstill, 2014.

Pottenger, Francis M. *Pottenger's Cats: A Study in Nutrition*. Lemon Grove, CA: Price-Pottenger Nutrition Foundation, 1983.

Raine Study: Western Australia Pregnancy Cohort. Studying 2,900 pregnant women and the health of their children over 27 years. Over 300 published studies available at http://rainestudy.production1.claritycommunications.com.au/research-findings/publications.

Reiter, R.J., et al. "Melatonin and the Circadian System: Contributions to Successful Female Reproduction." *Fertility and Sterility* 102, no. 2 (2014): 321–28. doi:10.1016/j.fertnstert.2014.06.014.

Ross, J.A., J.D. Potter, et al. "Maternal Exposure to Potential Inhibitors of DNA Topoisomerase II and Infant Leukemia (United States): A Report from the Children's Cancer Group." *Cancer Causes and Control* 7, no. 6 (1996): 581–90.

Rushing, Reece. "Reproductive Roulette: Declining Reproductive Health, Dangerous Chemicals, and a New Way Forward." *Center for American Progress*, July 21, 2009. www.americanprogress.org/issues/women/reports/2009/07/21/6431/reproductive-roulette.

Sender, R., S. Fuchs, and R. Milo. "Revised Estimates for the Number of Human and Bacteria Cells in the Body." *PLoS Biology* 14, no. 8 (2016). doi:10.1101/036103.

Singer, Katie. "Fertility Awareness, Food, and Night-Lighting." *Wise Traditions in Food, Farming and the Healing Arts*. Weston A. Price Foundation, Spring 2004.

Sonnenburg, Erida D., et al. "Diet-Induced Extinctions in the Gut Microbiota Compound Over Generations." *Nature* 529, no. 7585 (2016): 212–15. doi:10.1038/nature16504.

Strick, R., P.L. Strissel, et al. "Dietary Bioflavonids Induce Cleavage in the MLL Gene and May Contribute to Infant Leukemia." *Proceedings of the National Academy of Sciences* 97, no. 9 (2000): 4790–95.

Strom, B.L., et al. "Exposure to Soy-Based Formula in Infancy and Endocrinological and Reproductive Outcomes in Young Adulthood." *JAMA* 286, no. 7 (2001): 2402–403.

"The Canadian Organic Market Is Worth $4.7 Billion Per Year," *Globe and Mail*, Friday, September 16, 2016.

Tuan, Rocky S., ed. *Birth Defects Research Part C: Embryo Today: Reviews* 108, no. 2 (2016).

Vilella, Felipe, et al. "Hsa-miR-30d, Secreted by the Human Endometrium, Is Taken Up by the Pre-implantation Embryo and Might Modify Its Transcriptome." *Development* 142, no. 18 (2015): 3210–21. doi:10.1242/dev.124289.

Vilela, M.L., E. Willingham, J. Buckley, et al. "Endocrine Disruptors and Hypospadias: Role of Genistein and the Fungicide Vinclozolin." *Urology* 70, no. 3 (2007): 618–21.

Weed, Susun. *Wise Woman Herbal for the Childbearing Year*. Woodstock, NY: Ash Tree, 1996.

White, L. "Association of High Midlife Tofu Consumption with Accelerated Brain Aging." Plenary Session #8: Cognitive Function, The Third International Soy Symposium, Program, November 1999, 26.

Whitley, E., et al. "Paternal Age in Relation to Offspring Intelligence in the West of Scotland Twenty-07 Prospective Cohort Study." *PLoS One* 7, no. 12 (2012). doi:10.1371/journal.pone.0052112.

Wohl, M., and P. Gorwood. "Paternal Ages Below or Above 35 Years Old Are Associated with a Different Risk of Schizophrenia in the Offspring." *European Psychiatry* 22, no. 1 (2007): 22–26. doi:10.1016/j.eurpsy.2006.08.007.

Photo Credits

About the Photographers

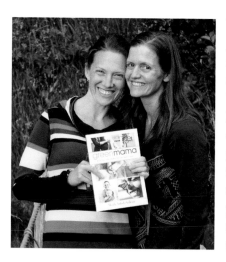

Vanessa Zises Filley is an award-winning photographer and mixed-media artist. This is her second book in the Green Mama series. More about her and her work can be found at **vanessafilley.com**. **Roxanne Engstrom** travels, volunteers, mothers, captures the humanity in each of us — people of every ethnicity and culture — through images and storytelling. Find her at **hawaimages.com**. **Cassie Rodgers** is a professional photographer and a pre/post-natal yoga specialist. See more of her work at **anandawithin.com**.

Vanessa Filley: 13, 23, 28, 31, 33, 38, 47, 54, 55, 65, 72, 99, 100, 106, 113, 115, 116, 128, 133, 191

Roxanne Engstrom: 14, 16, 19, 24, 146, 149, 150, 200, 209

Cassie Rodgers: 6, 12, 74, 93, 140, 153, 154, 155, 174–77, 178, 199

Manda Aufochs Gillespie: 20, 123, 124, 126, 159, 168, 185, 205, 214

Anna Lau: 165

Jan Sonnenmair (www.sonnenmair.com): 217

Index